While AIDS is a threat to people of any age, statistics show that because of their sexual activity, young people are the most at risk. How can we teach young people to protect themselves from the AIDS epidemic? Is there any effective means of prevention? What is the truth about AIDS and its transmission?

Writing a "book of hope for parents," Clif Cartland tells how *You Can Protect Yourself and Your Family From AIDS*. He draws upon the latest medical research and interviews with kids and parents to provide you with the guidance you need to communicate openly with your children. His reliable, straightforward counsel includes:

- what the schools are telling your children about AIDS (or soon will be)

- a discussion of what AIDS is and how it affects the body

- the counsel kids want to hear from their parents regarding AIDS and sexual activity

- the best way to avoid contracting AIDS

- what kids "know" about AIDS and how it is transmitted

- ways young people can experience intimacy without sexual activity

YOU CAN PROTECT YOURSELF AND YOUR FAMILY FROM AIDS

Clif Cartland

Power Books

FLEMING H. REVELL COMPANY
OLD TAPPAN, NEW JERSEY

ISBN 0-8007-5262-7

Copyright © 1987 by Clif Cartland
Published by the Fleming H. Revell Company
Old Tappan, New Jersey 07675
Printed in the United States of America

CONTENTS

A Fearful Nation ... Looking for Answers ... Some-
body's Got to Do Something ... It Can't Happen to Me ...
A High Risk Generation ... Why You Bought This Book
... The Road Ahead

Accepting Responsibility ... What I Found in My Search
... Hard Facts and Fragile Figures ... No Vaccine ... No
Cure ... The Cause of AIDS Discovered ... The Body's
Immune System ... Antibodies in the Blood ... The
AIDS Test ... Effects of the Virus ... ARC ... AIDS ...
Damage to the Nervous System ... How Is AIDS Trans-
mitted? ... Increasing Risk to Heterosexuals ... How the
Virus Is *Not* Spread ... Can AIDS Be Spread by Kissing?
... HIV in Semen and Blood ... The Risks of Anal Sex ...
Oral Sex ... The Number of Sexual Partners ... Intrave-
nous Drug Users ... Mother Can Infect the Newborn ...
Information Isn't Enough

Contents

This book is gratefully dedicated to

* My wife, Faith, my children, and grandchildren, who provide unrestrained support and encouragement, and keep me in touch with the wonder and the work of family life.
* Del Burnett, my dear friend, who cares enough to help me keep my priorities straight.
* Carlene Pote, both friend and co-worker, who labored with me through the many stages of this book.
* The doctors and parents who critiqued the manuscript and offered so many helpful suggestions.
* The dedicated people who search untiringly for more insight into this dreaded disease, and those doctors and nurses who treat people with AIDS.
* And last, but by no means least, those people whose hopes and dreams have been so cruelly interrupted by AIDS. May their tragedy help to encourage others to practice wise, protective behavior.

A portion of the royalties from this book go to providing care for people with AIDS whose financial resources are depleted.

PREFACE

The information contained in this book is based on the *United States Surgeon General's Report on AIDS*, released in October 1986, as well as on other medical information available as of June 1987.

While information and research are increasing daily, the basic health precautions necessary to protect yourself and your family from AIDS are not likely to change from those outlined in this book.

However, intense concern and extensive research are producing a constant flow of new medical information about AIDS. You are urged to direct questions about AIDS or any other medical subject to your own physician.

Your local or state public health office and the National AIDS Hotline (1-800-342-AIDS) can also provide you with a list of sources of the latest medical information on AIDS.

This book is offered for information purposes only, and is not intended to supplant medical advice, diagnosis, or treatment by a personal physician.

I'm not a medical doctor. I'm a concerned parent. I heard the Surgeon General say that parents ought to be talking to their kids about AIDS.

I knew he was right, but I also knew that wouldn't be easy. I've written about families and family concerns for years. I've been editor in chief of a family magazine. But I needed help on this tough subject, so I set out to find out *what* parents ought to say, and *how* to say it.

The result is, I believe, a book you can trust—a source book on AIDS written in language you and your kids can understand. But this is something more than a book of cold, hard facts. As I worked on the book, I began to have a deepened, more compassionate concern for a young person's search for intimacy. As you read, I hope you can begin to feel greater compassion and understanding for your own kids.

Talking to kids about sex is tough. Talking to kids about AIDS is even tougher. The natural tendency is to play the parent role to the fullest, to talk down to them.

I've tried to provide caring parents like you with some ways to come alongside kids and talk face-to-face about hard facts and tough decisions in a kindly, compassionate way. Kids *can* protect themselves from AIDS, and they need to have that fact reinforced by their parents.

If this book helps to increase understanding between parents and young people, if lines of communication can be opened about AIDS, sexuality, and the perils and promises of growing up, it will have served its purpose. And this parent/researcher/writer will have been richly rewarded.

STATEMENT OF
C. EVERETT KOOP, M.D., Sc.D.
SURGEON GENERAL
U.S. PUBLIC HEALTH SERVICE

AND

DEPUTY ASSISTANT SECRETARY OF HEALTH
DEPARTMENT OF HEALTH AND
HUMAN SERVICES

BEFORE THE
SELECT COMMITTEE ON CHILDREN, YOUTH,
AND FAMILIES
U.S. HOUSE OF REPRESENTATIVES
JUNE 18, 1987

Statement

Mr. Chairman and members of the Committee:

I welcome the opportunity to appear before you on an issue of the utmost concern to me—teenagers and AIDS. As a practicing pediatric surgeon for over forty years, the welfare of children and young adults has always been foremost in my thoughts.

Adolescents and preadolescents are those with behavior we wish to especially influence because of their vulnerability when they are exploring their own sexuality and perhaps experimenting with drugs. Teenagers often consider themselves immortal, and these young people may be putting themselves at great risk.

Extent of Risk

Some data provide information about the risk American teenagers have for becoming infected with the AIDS virus.

- About 2.5 million teenagers are affected by sexually transmitted diseases each year. In the United States, the most frequent mode of transmission for the AIDS virus is through sexual contact.

- American teenage females experience about 1 million unplanned pregnancies each year. These data indicate not only the extent to which teenagers are sexually active, but also the extent to which they might transmit the virus perinatally.

- More than 80 percent of unmarried males and 70 percent of unmarried females self-report that they have experienced intercourse at least once by age 20.

- About 1 percent of American high school seniors self-report having ever used heroin, 16.7 percent report having ever used cocaine, and 23.4 percent report having ever used stimulants; all of these drugs can be taken intravenously. Although teenagers generally do not inject drugs, those who do and share needles are at increased risk for infection with the AIDS virus.

Since the most frequent mode of transmission for the AIDS virus is through sexual contact, it is clear that teenagers are very much at risk. To date, only 1 percent of all AIDS cases has occurred among persons under age 20 (most of whom were infected by transfusion or perinatal transmission); about 21 percent of all cases have been diagnosed in the 20–29 age group. Since the time between infection with the AIDS virus and onset of symptoms may be several years, some proportion of those aged 20–29 who have been diagnosed with AIDS were most likely infected as teenagers.

Although these data demonstrate that many teenagers are at risk of becoming infected, most teenagers do not believe they are. Indeed, a random sample of 860 Massachusetts youth aged 16–19 revealed that while 70 percent reported they were sexually active, only 15 percent of them reported changing their sexual behavior because of concern about contracting AIDS; and only 20 percent of those who changed their behavior used effective methods.

I believe that education about AIDS should begin at home so that children can grow up knowing the behavior to avoid to protect themselves from exposure to the AIDS virus. This behavior should be reinforced in the schools. I recommend that parents establish the biological and moral bases for sexual activity early so that when their children become teenagers they will make decisions about their sexual behavior that can eliminate the risk of getting AIDS.

Most teenagers want to know more about AIDS. In a public poll conducted in the fall of 1986, 86 percent of parents questioned agreed that sex education courses should be taught in school; and, of those, 95 percent agreed that such courses should teach 12-year-olds about the danger of AIDS. The nation's system of public and private schools can play a vital role in assuring that all young people rapidly understand the nature of the epidemic they face, and specific actions they can take to protect themselves from becoming infected, especially during their teenage years, as well as when they become adults. We believe that: (1) the scope and content of AIDS education should be determined locally and should be consistent with parental values; (2) that information developed by the federal government to educate young people about AIDS should encourage responsible sexual behavior—based on fidelity, commitment, and maturity, placing sexuality within the context of marriage; (3) any health information provided by the federal government that might be used in schools should teach that children should not engage in sex before they are ready to marry.

These principles, approved by the president and cited by Secretary Bowen in the AIDS information plan, will be followed to the fullest extent in the development of any federal educational material that might be used in schools.

Statement

According to information gathered during the winter of 1986, 40 of the nation's 73 largest school districts were providing education about AIDS; 24 more were planning such education. Of the districts that provided AIDS education, 90 percent provided it during 10th grade, 63 percent provided it during 7th grade, and 60 percent provided it during 9th grade. I agree with Mayor Koch of New York that, in addition to not using IV drugs, abstinence from promiscuous sexual activity or monogamy is the only way for adolescents to avoid getting AIDS.

School Health Education

Because AIDS is a fatal disease, and because educating young people about the risks of becoming infected through sexual contact can be controversial, health education programs about AIDS should be developed as quickly as possible, with parental participation, by all school systems. In each community, parents, representatives of the school board, school administrators and faculty, school health services, local medical societies, the local health department, students (at appropriate grades), religious organizations, and other relevant community organizations should be involved in planning and periodically assessing programs of school health education about AIDS.

It is most important that teenagers receive education that specifically would enable them to understand and avoid behaviors associated with transmission of the AIDS virus. A single pamphlet, a single filmstrip, a single lecture about AIDS will not be sufficient. Similarly, education about the biology of the virus, the symptoms of

15

the disease, or the social and economic consequences of the epidemic will do little to influence its spread. Programs need to be designed specifically to help teenagers adopt the kind of behavior which will keep them from contracting this disease. It is especially important that school sex education programs emphasize to teenagers the need to refrain from sexual intercourse until they are ready to establish a mutually faithful, monogamous relationship. I believe that it is possible to focus on preadolescent youngsters and produce a generation of teenagers who will remain abstinent until they develop a mature, monogamous relationship.

Outlined below are some of the efforts being undertaken by agencies of the Public Health Service that focus on the problem of AIDS among teenagers. All of these programs are meant to assist local organizations in establishing their own prevention programs.

Centers for Disease Control (CDC)

In fiscal year 1987, CDC will work with national educational organizations and state and local departments of education to develop information that may help schools across the nation implement effective education to prevent the spread of AIDS.

National Organizations

CDC will award cooperative agreements to about 7 national organizations that represent parents, school boards, school administrators, teachers, medical professionals, church groups, and other important professional and voluntary health and education organizations. In addition, 4 awards will be made to national organizations that respectively can develop AIDS education programs for minorities, mainly Black and Hispanic; develop programs for college students, and develop programs so that colleges of education deliver inservice and preservice training to teachers so that they may be able to provide effective education about AIDS. Finally, 1 cooperative agreement will be awarded to a national organization that can help all 56 state and territorial departments of education to assist schools in their respective jurisdictions provide effective education about AIDS.

State and Local Departments of Education

In 1987, CDC plans to award cooperative agreements to 10 state departments of education and 12 local departments of education that serve jurisdictions with the highest cumulative incidence of AIDS. Nineteen states that had reported 200 or more diagnosed AIDS cases, and 18 cities that reported 150 or more cases by the last day of 1986, will be eligible for these awards. The purpose of these agreements is to provide fiscal support and technical assistance to help state and local education departments implement intensive education about AIDS principally for school-age youth, in and out of school.

Training and Demonstration Projects

In the fall of 1987, CDC will provide additional support to each of 3 local and 1 state departments of education to also establish training and demonstration projects. Support consequently will be provided to at least 300 local and state department of education personnel from other jurisdictions to attend these projects and to receive assistance for implementing effective school health education about AIDS in their own areas.

Development and Dissemination of Educational Curricula and Materials

Technical and limited fiscal assistance will be provided to help relevant private sector organizations develop, evaluate, and disseminate a variety of scientifically accurate and effective educational materials for school-age populations. CDC has established a subfile on *School Health Education about AIDS* within its Combined Health Information Database system, an annotated computerized bibliography that can be easily accessed. The file describes age-appropriate AIDS education materials, curricula, programs, research, and resources that have already been developed and how to acquire them. A compendium of selected resources will be published and disseminated periodically.

Research and Evaluation

CDC will compile, synthesize, apply, and disseminate the results of research that could improve the effectiveness of school health education to prevent the spread of AIDS; and will assist national, state, and local agencies to evaluate and consequently improve their program efforts.

Alcohol, Drug Abuse, and Mental Health Administration (ADAMHA)

An example of research on AIDS conducted by the National Institute on Drug Abuse that focuses on teenagers is an AIDS demonstration/training project entitled

AIDS Prevention Among High Risk Adolescent Populations. This 1-year project, to be awarded in fiscal year
1987, is designed to identify specific subsets of adolescent
populations at the highest risk for AIDS and develop
strategies for reaching, communicating AIDS information
to, and counseling them. After an initial data collection
effort, experts will be brought together to review what has
been learned regarding informing and counseling adolescents. A guide will be developed based upon clinical
experience and research. A training program will be
tested and developed, also.

In addition, a group of young people who appear to be
at high risk for contracting AIDS are adolescents who are
homeless and living on the streets or in shelters. The
National Institute of Mental Health, in collaboration with
other PHS components and the Administration on Children, Youth, and Families, has organized a workshop on
June 22–23 on AIDS and Adolescents in Crisis to discuss
prevention, intervention, and treatment for this high-risk
group.

Health Resources and Services Administration (HRSA)

Two of the four AIDS Service Demonstration Program
grant projects administered by HRSA have components
on adolescent prevention/education:

- The New York State Department of Health has
  awarded a 3-year subcontract to the Institute for the
  Protection of Lesbian and Gay Youth. HRSA and
  Robert Wood Johnson Foundation grant funds are
  assisting them in developing AIDS/HIV infection ma-

terials and teaching strategies for adolescents, and provide direct counseling services at a "drop-in center" to high-risk adolescents, some of whom are homeless, and many of whom are or have been involved with prostitution.

- The Los Angeles Department of Health, AIDS Program Office, has 3 subcontracts, supported with HRSA service demonstration funds, that reach adolescents in Black and Hispanic communities in Central, South Central, and East Los Angeles. The Watts Health Foundation and the Minority AIDS Project are involved with risk reduction education programs, outreach and referral services targeted to minority youth. El Centro Human Services organization is attempting to reach adolescents at risk, particularly IV drug abusers, in a predominantly Mexican American area of Los Angeles.

National Institutes of Health (NIH)

The National Institute of Child Health and Human Development (NICHD) plans to support several research initiatives that are expected to provide valuable information related to AIDS and teenagers. NICHD will request grant applications for projects that would describe and explain the behavior patterns that put teenagers at risk of exposure to HIV and for projects to study the process by which individuals incorporate concerns about sexually transmitted diseases and AIDS into decisions to be sexually active and to use or not use contraceptives. The institute also plans to support seminars concerning AIDS for obstetricians, gynecologists, and pediatricians. These seminars, planned for the fall of 1987, will provide information for further dissemination to other medical providers, patients, and educators.

Conclusion

Although 148 cases of AIDS have been reported to date among young people aged 13 to 19, there is hope that:

- AIDS is not common yet among adolescents.

- We know a lot and can know more about how to effectively work with this age group.

- For many of our teenagers, this would be a preventive intervention, especially in very young teens. And after all, it is easier to prevent some behavior than to change it.

- AIDS may give us the impetus to deal knowledgeably and effectively with a whole range of health-related behaviors in adolescents.

Let me conclude with a quote from the *Surgeon General's Report on AIDS:*

> Those of us who are parents, educators, and community leaders, indeed all adults, cannot disregard this responsibility to educate our young. The need is critical and the price of neglect is high. The lives of our young people depend on our fulfilling our responsibility.

PART 1
Understanding AIDS

You run into a lot of so-called AIDS experts these days. Everybody seems to know *something* about AIDS. But everybody's "facts" can be very confusing.

In the pages ahead you'll find solid, documented information about AIDS. This information has been brought together, not to help you win an argument over coffee with your friends, but to help you protect yourself and your family from AIDS.

Read it carefully. Read it slowly. *Reread it* if necessary. Protection begins with knowing the facts.

1

First Steps to Protection

The doctors were puzzled—troubled was closer to the truth. Here were the medical histories of five young men, each from the Los Angeles area, each with the same kind of very rare lung infection.

Sometimes this kind of infection was seen in transplant patients, or in people receiving chemotherapy. But none of these men fit that description.

The youngest of the group was twenty-nine, the oldest only thirty-six. They did not know one another and had no common contacts. Yet they all had Pneumocystis carinii pneumonia (new-mo-SIS-tis kar-IN-e-eye noo-MOAN-e-uh).

The twenty-nine-year-old had been admitted to the hospital in February, and died in March. Another man, thirty-three years old, had battled a fever for two months before being admitted to the hospital in March for treatment of pneumonia. He died early in May.

The others were still alive, but their stories were similar. They, like the other two, were sexually active homosexuals.[1] (Two of the five reported having "various partners.") They had all been healthy; then came the fever and the pneumonia.

A team of medical specialists had considered several possible causes. Could they have caught the disease from a sexual partner? At the time, the answer seemed to be no. Other possibilities were considered, and tests were made, but there were no clear answers to their questions, and their concern was mounting.

Five doctors from the School of Medicine at the University of California, Los Angeles, and another from Cedars-Sinai Hospital, Los Angeles, joined in filing a report on these five young men with the federal Centers for Disease Control (CDC) in Atlanta, Georgia.

Analysts for the CDC called this occurrence "unusual," but found it difficult to reach "definite conclusions ... because of the lack of published data."[2] That very first CDC report on the condition that was soon to become known as AIDS (acquired immune deficiency syndrome) was published in June 1981.

By the end of that year, the number of people with fully developed AIDS[3] had grown to about 250. Today, in the

---

1. A *homosexual* is a person who is sexually attracted to persons of the *same* sex. Homosexual men are sometimes called "gay." Homosexual women are known as Lesbians.
2. *Morbidity and Mortality Weekly Report*, June 5, 1981, published by United States Department of Health and Human Services, Public Health Service, Centers for Disease Control, Atlanta, Georgia.
3. Throughout this book, the term *fully developed AIDS* is used to indicate the condition in which the body's immune system is being destroyed, reducing its ability to fight off infection and cancers. (See chapter 2 for a more detailed explanation.)

United States alone there have been more than 35,000 reported cases of people with fully developed AIDS. Over 20,000 of those have died, and the rest are not expected to survive.

In the United States, between a million and a million and a half people have already been infected with the virus and are now capable of infecting others.

Dr. Jonathan Mann, head of the World Health Organization (WHO) AIDS program estimates that there are more than one hundred thousand cases of fully developed AIDS worldwide. In addition, WHO estimates that between five and ten million people throughout the world are infected with the virus.

This is an epidemic that should sober the most optimistic among us.

A Fearful Nation

If you can put your ear close to the heart of America you will hear the sounds of yet another epidemic. It is not a mysterious clinical disease, yet it paralyzes the soul. This epidemic of the spirit has been called "afrAIDS,"[4] and it seems to be infecting more and more people. In fact, 38 percent of Americans—more than ninety-two million people—say they are very concerned about AIDS as a problem to *their own health,* according to an NBC/ *Wall Street Journal* poll.

We were just beginning to believe that medicine was a match for almost any malady. Diseases that were disas-

---

4. This term was used in the *New Republic*, October 14, 1985.

trous only decades ago had all but disappeared. At least some of the sting was gone from the dreaded word *cancer*. Given time, talent, and telethons we would soon lick the other diseases.

Then came AIDS, this frightening *new* disease.

At first it didn't affect us. It was a homosexual disease, we thought. We were curious but not too concerned.

Next came the reports of intravenous or IV (injected into the vein) drug abusers contracting AIDS. Then people with hemophilia.[5] And the children of mothers with the virus. Then people whose only common ground was the fact that they had received blood transfusions.

We were beginning to see that a disease we thought only infected "others" could now be a risk to us. And with that realization came the fears.

Looking for Answers

AIDS is a disease that produces far more questions than ready, simple answers. And that troubles us, for fear thrives in an atmosphere of uncertainty.

We want answers—clear, unequivocal answers. We want so much to calm our fears or confirm our suspicions that we're often willing to believe almost anyone whose information sounds reliable. But only the facts—carefully gathered and clearly presented—can calm those fears.

---

5. *Hemophilia* is a disease in which males are born with a bleeding tendency due to poor clot formation. They often hemorrhage or bleed uncontrollably after minor injuries, and require special transfusions to stop or prevent bleeding.

That is what I have attempted to do throughout this book. Every medical statement has been thoroughly checked by AIDS researchers and physicians who provide medical care for AIDS victims every day.

People have said to me, "I want to believe that my family and I are not in danger, but when it comes to my kids or my grandkids ... I'm still not sure what's safe."

Despite assurances that there is no danger in casual contact with AIDS victims, we sometimes choose to believe misinformation rather than the facts.

Some of us panic at the thought of a child with AIDS going to school with our child. Others won't eat where we suspect that the cook or waiter may be homosexual.

Careful, conscientious researchers tell us that these fears, and a host of others like them, are absolutely baseless. Yet the fears persist.

Life is so precious and our fears are so much a part of us that it is difficult to hear the truth. But we must. The simple truth, the truth that could set us free from fear, is that *millions of us are at no risk whatsoever of contracting AIDS if we continue to maintain a mutually faithful, monogamous sexual relationship. Millions more of us could eliminate the possibility of future infection by changing our sexual practices.*

"Somebody's Got to Do Something!"

Sometimes our fears make us lash out at those we blame for the AIDS epidemic. We still think of it as "a gay

29

disease." "If it wasn't for those homosexuals," we say, ignoring the fact that, worldwide, as many women as men are infected with the virus; ignoring the fact that in every other part of the world the primary method of transmission of AIDS is through *heterosexual*[6] sex activity.

As the AIDS death toll mounts and the epidemic spreads, our fears and frustrations give way to a call for action. After all, "somebody *has* to do *something*." But the rush to "do something," the popular political answers, the campaign oratory, must always be carefully weighed against the counsel of those whose lives are dedicated to finding *real* and lasting answers to the AIDS dilemma: the public health workers, the medical profession, and the researchers.

The lives of your family and mine will not be protected by political answers. No quarantines or overnight massive testing programs can ferret out the real culprits in the AIDS epidemic.

The real culprits are us. We must all embrace the liberating yet bound-to-be painful truth, that our national fascination with "sex with whomever I want, whenever I want" must give way to a renewed commitment to faithfulness and fidelity. And no amount of political action can bring that about.

On a more human, more compassionate level, we must not ignore the fact that people with fully developed AIDS, *whoever they are*, are people whose lives and dreams have been shattered. Often they are kept alive by sheer

---

6. A *heterosexual* is a person who is sexually attracted to persons of the *opposite* sex.

courage. Instead of our caution and contempt, they deserve our care and compassion.

"It Can't Happen to Me"

There is yet a third epidemic, one that is perhaps the most difficult to battle. It threatens to destroy our young and diminish our bright hopes for the future. I call it the "evAIDS"[7] epidemic—evading the hard truth that to be sexually active is to risk contracting AIDS.

EvAIDS is particularly strong among the young. Enjoying freedom from parental constraint, the first breath of a life without limits, the young have no stomach for what we adults call "raw reality." To them, the flippant "It won't happen to me" is not so much a response to AIDS as it is a statement of wild, untainted hope. "It *can't* happen to me. How can it?"

The truth is that it *can*.

A High Risk Generation

In discussing the AIDS epidemic the Surgeon General said, "All of our young people are now at *high risk*. They are exploring their sexuality (heterosexual and homosexual) and perhaps experimenting with drugs.

"How they live out their sexuality over a long period of time will determine whether our society can survive this devastating disease or not."[8]

---

7. The spelling mistake is intentional in order to make a point.
8. From the *United States Surgeon General's Report on AIDS*, October 1986.

Sexual activity among the young is not the exception. It has become almost the rule. In a *People* magazine survey of teen sex, 57 percent of high school students and 79 percent of college students polled were already sexually active.

The same survey found that the overall age at which teenagers first had sexual intercourse was 16.9.[9]

In a poll of early adolescents conducted by the Search Institute, 15 percent of seventh graders (twelve-year-olds), 17 percent of eighth graders, and 20 percent of ninth graders reported having sexual intercourse ("making love" or "going all the way" as they choose to call it) one or more times.[10]

In late 1986, Louis Harris and Associates conducted a nationwide poll for the Planned Parenthood Federation on teenagers' views of sex, pregnancy, and birth control. That survey showed that approximately three out of every ten teenagers (28 percent), ages twelve to seventeen, say they have had sexual intercourse.

The proportion increases with age, from 4 percent of the twelve-year-olds and 10 percent of the thirteen-year-olds up to 46 percent of the sixteen-year-olds and 57 percent of the seventeen-year-olds.

According to this survey, more than half of all teenagers have had sexual intercourse by their seventeenth year.

These representative teens were also asked what they felt was the "right age" for a person to start having sexual intercourse. The median age given was eighteen. Only one-quarter said sixteen or younger.

---

9. Reported in *People* magazine, April 13, 1987.
10. Peter Benson, Arthur Johnson, and Dorothy Williams, *The Quicksilver Years* (New York: Harper & Row Publishers, 1986).

But 78 percent of those teenagers also said that they believe most teens in their school or neighborhood don't wait until then, but start having sexual intercourse earlier than the "right age."[11]

Why You Bought This Book

When we see these kinds of statistics, adults too can be overcome by evAIDS. And that's understandable. Some of us may suspect that our failure to care, our failure to communicate, and our failure to discipline is coming back to haunt us at the very point in the lives of our young when we are losing our ability to control their behavior.

Some of us are sure those sexually active young people belong to somebody else—not us.

If they *are* ours, we may not want to hear about it. Or, in the face of the truth, we say through our tears, "Don't ever let your father know."

It isn't easy to be a parent. You may feel as if you are up to your armpits in pressures and responsibilities—any one of which is more demanding than you had ever imagined. Then along comes this AIDS thing. . . .

You bought this book because you're serious about being the right kind of parent. Through the darkness of this AIDS epidemic, I believe you will find new depths of family openness and trust.

This book is about a painful subject, but I want it to be a book of hope. I've written it with these firm, abiding convictions:

---

11. Reported in *American Teens Speak: Sex, Myths, TV and Birth Control.* Conducted for the Planned Parenthood Federation of America, Inc.

- Almost every parent wants to do his or her best for their child, no matter how many times they've "blown it" in the past.
- Most broken parent/child relationships can be renewed if the parent will make the effort—or *efforts*—with patience and a willingness to listen.
- The fear of AIDS we all face gives parents an ideal opportunity to talk openly with their child.
- Young people want to have their parents talk about sex and AIDS in an atmosphere where a young person's thoughts are listened to and every question is taken seriously.
- Our young deserve nothing less than the best scientific, most honest information about AIDS and the ways in which it is transmitted. In this book you may find concepts and words that are difficult, even painful, to say. There has been no intent to be daring or shocking. But straight talk is necessary if kids are ever going to understand.

The Road Ahead

In the *People* magazine survey, conducted by New York-based Audits and Surveys, more than 95 percent of sexually active high school and college students polled knew that AIDS could be spread heterosexually; nevertheless, only 26 percent of high school students and 15 percent of college students surveyed had changed their sexual behavior.

It is clear that the stark figures of the AIDS epidemic alone are not enough to change the sexual activities of many young people. After all, sex can sometimes feel like love, and physical closeness can seem like the intimacy we all want so desperately.

The emotional needs of the young are real—and so demanding. The answers sex seems to offer feel so right that many are willing to play the odds, to risk the future for the pleasure of the present.

Most of us know that feeling, and we have come to realize that changing our behavior is almost always difficult. We also know what it is like to violate our best intentions. And at times most of us have felt the satisfaction of doing what we wanted so deeply to do—but weren't sure we could hold on.

Writing this book has made me face my own personal frailties—and my continuing struggle to be an effective, caring parent.

As you read, I hope you will be aware of your frailties in the sense that in the intimate matters of the heart, most of us are really children only slightly grown up.

If you can keep that in mind, you'll be able to proceed with compassion and understanding. Imagine as you read that you're hearing your young people say:

> Please be patient. Don't prejudge me by your moral standards. Stick with me when I don't meet those standards. I'm still worth loving and saving.
>
> Love me, even when you don't *like* me. Trust me. I need to know you're with me. If intimacy isn't sleeping around, please *show me what it is.* I need to know.

2

What Parents Need to Know About AIDS

When it comes to understanding AIDS, many of us today are just about where the doctors were in 1981 when the disease was first discovered.

We are confused—and concerned.

In just a few years medical science has put major pieces of this disturbing puzzle together. We need to be able to do the same thing.

What the experts know, *we* need to know. We also need to know what questions they have so we can protect ourselves and our families.

Accepting Responsibility

Some months ago, all I knew about AIDS was what I read in the papers and occasional magazine articles. Then in the fall of 1986 the *Surgeon General's Report on AIDS* was released.

This report took me beyond the newspaper stories. It was thorough and thoughtful—developed, Dr. Koop stated, after consulting with "the best medical and scientific experts this country can offer."[1]

There was something else Dr. Koop said in his report that struck a responsive chord:

"Those of us who are parents, educators, and community leaders, indeed all adults, cannot disregard [our] responsibility to educate our young [about AIDS]."

I knew I couldn't answer for educators and community leaders, but I am *a parent*, and if I had a responsibility to educate the young, I had to know more about this disease—and how to talk to kids about it.

With the *Surgeon General's Report on AIDS* as a foundation, I began gathering every other bit of printed information I could find: books, pamphlets, medical journals, press releases. I sometimes checked as many as five and six different sources for information on the same subject, looking for the clearest, most authoritative answer. Sometimes I read for hours to find a single word that made a statement more understandable to me.

Then medical doctors who work daily with people who have fully developed AIDS read everything I had written about the disease. They made corrections and suggestions. They directed me to medical journals for still more data. And finally they agreed that the material was medically accurate.

Parents read the same material for clarity, and offered their suggestions. Other physicians and researchers read the final manuscript for accuracy just before publication.

The result is one parent's search for the facts about AIDS; one parent's attempt to go beyond the things he

---

1. From the *Surgeon General's Report on AIDS*.

thought he knew about AIDS; one parent's attempt to get ready to talk with his own family with a feeling of assurance.

I can't stress too strongly the need to read—and *reread*—this chapter slowly and carefully. Feel free to write notes or questions in the margin.

Then ask your spouse or another adult friend to read the chapter, so that the two of you can talk about it together. This will help make the information clearer and make you more comfortable in sharing it with your kids.

What I Found in My Search

In the early 1980s most people with AIDS were in New York City, San Francisco, and Los Angeles. Most of them were homosexuals, intravenous[2] drug abusers, and persons with hemophilia.

Within five years the disease had begun to move from major cities to small towns and even rural areas. AIDS cases have been reported in all fifty states. By 1991, according to the Centers for Disease Control (CDC), four out of five new persons with AIDS (80 percent) will be found outside New York and California. And more and more of those victims will be *heterosexuals*.

According to the U.S. Surgeon General, it is conservatively estimated that there are between a million and a million and a half Americans who have been infected with the deadly AIDS virus, and are capable of infecting their sex partners.

---

2. Also called IV. Intravenous drug abusers inject drugs into a vein.

AIDS cases have now been reported in 132 countries.

By 1991 possibly as many Americans will die in one year from AIDS in the United States alone as died in ten years of the Vietnam war—and they will be men and women from roughly the same young age group.

Hard Facts and Fragile Futures

People who are referred to as "having AIDS" are struggling with life-threatening illnesses. They are in the final stages of a series of health problems caused by a virus that can be passed from one person to another primarily during sexual intercourse, through the sharing of intravenous drug needles and syringes used for "shooting" illegal drugs, or from receiving transfusions of contaminated blood. (More specific details on kinds of activities through which the virus is transmitted will be found later in this chapter and in chapter 3.)

A person infected with the virus may not show any symptoms, or resemble the hospitalized people with AIDS whose pictures you have seen on television. We call that infected person a "healthy carrier." But even though there are no symptoms to indicate to the individual, a physician, or anyone else that they are infected, he or she:

1. is capable of transmitting the virus to someone else, and

2. will never be free from the virus.

The effects of the virus range from lying dormant in the body for years to causing death within months. Ten to 30 percent of people infected with the virus will have fully developed AIDS within five years. These percentages may change in the years ahead.

Dr. Anthony S. Fauci, director of the National Institute of Allergy and Infectious Diseases in Bethesda, Maryland, looked beyond that five-year point in a radio interview:

> You could have been infected with the virus years ago, still be living a healthy life, and get sick from it years from now.
>
> We know for sure that it can be as long as five to seven years [before symptoms show up]. It might even be as long as twelve to fifteen years.
>
> It appears that after five years, instead of leveling off, the percentage of those who develop the full-blown disease actually accelerates.

No Vaccine

Scientists are working to develop a safe, effective vaccine to protect against the AIDS virus. Progress is steady but slow. One vaccine has now been approved for testing.

But most researchers in this country and in France say that it will take until the end of the century before an effective vaccine will be available. To further complicate matters, several strains of HIV virus have been identified, and no one vaccine could protect against all the strains.

No Cure

"Once a person is infected [with the virus] he or she will never be cured," says Dr. Flossie Wong-Stall[3] of the National Cancer Institute.

Once people are diagnosed as having fully developed AIDS, 50 percent die within one year, and more than 95 percent die within two years. Only a handful survive longer than three years.

The average survival time of a person with fully developed AIDS is eighteen months from diagnosis to death.

The AIDS virus multiplies within the person's body cells. One hundred viruses become two hundred, two hundred become four hundred, and so on, destroying the body's natural immune system until it can no longer protect itself against germs and cancers.

A drug called AZT (azidothymidine—a-ZY-do-THIGH-mah-deen), known by the trade name Retrovir®, is now available to people with AIDS. AZT can alter the ability of the virus to multiply and it delays the deadly complications of AIDS. It does not get rid of the remaining virus, but it can prolong life.

"It seems as though [the disease] progresses at a slower rate. But it still progresses. Patients still die, even while they're getting AZT," reported Dr. Paul Volberding, an AIDS researcher at San Francisco General Hospital, in a radio interview.

---

3. Dr. Wong-Stall is Section Chief for Molecular Genetics of Hematopoietic Cells, in the Laboratory for Tumor Cell Biology of the National Cancer Institute.

The Cause of AIDS Discovered

In 1984, scientists at the National Cancer Institute were able to identify the cause of AIDS as one of the "human retroviruses." They were able to pinpoint a specific one. They called it the human T-lymphotropic (lim-fo-TRO-pic) virus type III, or more simply HTLV-III.

At about the same time, a closely related virus was found in studies at the Pasteur Institute in France. There it became known as the lymphadenopathy (lim-fah-den-OP-athy) associated virus or LAV. An international committee of scientists has decided to call the virus by the single common name human immunodeficiency (im-YUNE-oh-de-FISH-un-see) virus.

When we speak of the virus we should use the term HIV, the proper name for the virus. When we talk about someone having AIDS (or, as we have chosen to call it, fully developed AIDS), we are referring to the advanced symptoms and conditions caused by HIV, the virus.

The Body's Immune System

Our body has a natural immune system that helps us fight off infection.

When a germ or virus enters our body a certain kind of white blood cells called lymphocytes (LIM-fo-sites) produce substances that attack and destroy the invading germs.

HIV (the AIDS virus) attacks the body's immune system and actually becomes a permanent part of certain cells, particularly the T-lymphocytes.[4] There the virus remains temporarily harmless to the individual. However, it can still be passed on to infect someone else through direct semen-to-blood or blood-to-blood contact.

"[The virus] takes a free ride as long as it can," reports biologist Gary Nabel. "Then when the T-lymphocyte is about to do its [infection-fighting] job, the virus reproduces and kills the cell."[5] As the virus spreads it destroys more and more T-lymphocytes until the immune system is left with too few to ward off infection.

The HIV also attacks the central nervous system, including the brain cells.

Antibodies in the Blood

Typically, six to twelve weeks[6] after the virus enters the bloodstream, the body begins to produce a disease-fighting protein substance called antibodies. But these antibodies are not strong enough to eliminate the HIV.

The AIDS Test

A simple blood test is now available that can detect antibodies to the HIV virus. It does not test for the virus directly.

---

4. The "T" indicates that these lymphocytes mature in the thymus gland.
5. From a report by Gary Nabel on research he conducted with David Baltimore. Nabel and Baltimore are molecular biologists at the Whitehead Institute for Biomedical Research, Cambridge, Massachusetts.
6. Cases have been reported in which antibodies were not present in the blood of an infected individual until up to eight months after exposure to HIV.

The test is performed about eighty thousand times every working day. A new, clean needle is used to draw a small amount of blood from the arm for an Enzyme-Linked Immunosorbent Assay or ELISA (e-LIE-za) test.

If the result is positive (that is, antibodies to HIV are found in the blood), a second, more specific antibody test, called a Western blot test, is done.

If the second test shows a positive result, the person has been exposed to the virus and is infected.

If the test is negative, this *usually* means that the person has not been infected. However, the two types of tests mentioned above indicate only the presence of *antibodies* to HIV, and it takes six to twelve weeks after infection for antibodies to develop. If within that time period the person tested has had additional sexual activity, a negative test result does not guarantee that the person is free of the virus.

Recently, Abbott Laboratories applied to the U.S. Food and Drug Administration for approval to market a new blood test. Because this test directly indicates the presence of antigens to the AIDS virus, it may provide earlier detection of HIV infection.

It is of vital importance that any AIDS test be accompanied with counseling before and after testing. A person generally takes the test because of concerns caused by sexual activity or IV drug abuse. This makes it essential that the person understand the importance of changing sexual practices and eliminating high-risk behavior.

Effects of the Virus

It is suspected that more than 90 percent of those infected with HIV will begin to experience some immune system problems within five years after infection.

Once a person is infected, the effects of the virus differ. Some people will remain well, even though they are able to infect sexual partners.

ARC

For some people, infection results in AIDS-Related Complex (ARC). This is a name some scientists use to describe physical conditions that are generally less severe than fully developed AIDS. However, people do die from ARC.

Signs and symptoms of ARC may include the following:

- Extreme tiredness and loss of appetite sometimes accompanied by headache, dizziness, or light-headedness, lasting more than one month.

- Swollen or tender glands, with or without pain, in the neck, jaw, armpits, or groin, lasting more than one month.

- Skin rashes.

- Continued fever—body temperatures over 101 degrees for more than two weeks.

- Weight loss of more than ten pounds in a short time, which is not due to dieting or increased physical activity.

- Lack of resistance to infection.

- Heavy, continual cough (often dry) that is not from smoking or that has lasted too long to be a cold or flu (more than two weeks), often associated with fever and shortness of breath.

- Unexplained diarrhea, persisting more than two weeks.

- Progressive shortness of breath.

- Black and blue bruises or a bleeding tendency.

- Neurological impairments: sensory, motor, intellect, personality.

It is important to know that these are also signs and symptoms of many other diseases. A person with any of these symptoms should see a physician for evaluation.

AIDS

Only a qualified health professional should diagnose AIDS.

When a person has fully developed AIDS, more and more T-lymphocytes are being destroyed until the body's immune system cannot protect itself against germs and cancers that would normally not be able to gain a foothold. These are called "opportunistic diseases." They use the body's lowered resistance as an opportunity to infect and destroy the body.

Some symptoms of AIDS and these "opportunistic" infections may include a persistent cough and fever with shortness of breath or difficult breathing. These may be the symptoms of Pneumocystis carinii pneumonia. While the Pneumocystis carinii parasite is in the system of most humans, it usually causes no trouble or symptoms.

46

However, when the body's immune system is destroyed, the parasite causes the very destructive pneumonia to which a large number of people with AIDS succumb.

Infected individuals may also develop certain types of cancers such as Kaposi's sarcoma (KAP-oh-sees sar-COMB-uh). This cancer produces purplish blotches and bumps on or under the skin, inside the mouth, eyelids, nose, and rectum, and on internal organs. It is one of the visible and often disfiguring signs of fully developed AIDS.

Damage to the Nervous System

In many people the virus may also attack the nervous system early in the disease and cause damage to the brain.

This damage can also take years to develop. The symptoms may show up as memory loss, indifference, loss of coordination, partial paralysis, or other mental disorders.

Problems with the nervous system have been found in as many as 90 percent of people who die as a result of HIV-related conditions. Sometimes the virus causes significant problems with the central nervous system, even though there is no apparent damage to the immune system.

How Is AIDS Transmitted?

The virus is transmitted only through blood-to-blood or semen-to-blood contact. Most people with AIDS contract the disease through sexual activity (*see* pages 50-53 for more detailed information), contaminated blood left in needles and syringes being reused by IV drug abusers, the transfusion of untested blood products from an infected donor to a noninfected recipient,[7] and from an HIV-infected mother to her unborn child.

Increasing Risk to Heterosexuals

Although AIDS was first discovered among homosexuals, the disease is not the result of homosexuality, nor is it limited to homosexuals. In fact, *throughout the world, HIV is found almost equally in men and women.*

Dr. Robert Gallo of the National Cancer Institute has observed:

> There is nothing special about this virus by logic that should have said that this is a virus of homosexuals. We handled that question in that way in the beginning, but we never thought that there was anything that was special about homosexuals—only that they were the group in the Western hemisphere that had the most contact with the virus, and keeping mostly to themselves, it was confined to that population. Clearly the virus can go man-man, man-woman,

---

7. Since May 1985, all donated blood in the United States has been tested for HIV. Before that date, the AIDS virus was transmitted to some persons with hemophilia and others who received blood transfusions. As an extra precaution, most physicians are now more cautious in ordering transfusions.

woman-man, and I don't think there is a bit of interest in the mode of sex.[8]

In Africa AIDS is transmitted primarily by heterosexuals. Victims are equally divided between men and women. "You could have exactly the same condition in the United States and Europe five years from now," according to Dr. Robert Redfield of the Walter Reed Army Institute of Research in Washington, D.C.

Surgeon General Koop says, "While only four percent of AIDS patients today in the U.S. are heterosexual, we anticipate a rather sharp increase in the next four years."

Dr. Koop worries that as many as twenty-eight thousand heterosexual Americans not now infected with HIV may be suffering from fully developed AIDS in five years. "It's predicted on the basis of everything we know that, while AIDS will increase ninefold overall in the next five years, it will increase twentyfold among heterosexuals."

How the Virus Is *Not* Spread

HIV is not spread by casual, everyday kinds of contact, such as hugging, shaking hands, being sneezed on, or even sharing a soda.

The virus is very sensitive to temperature and to drying. It can survive for less than two hours outside the body. In normal household cleanup it is destroyed by

---

8. James I. Slaff, M.D., and John K. Brubaker, *The AIDS Epidemic* (New York: Warner Books, 1985).

1 part household bleach to 10 parts water[9]

Lysol

alcohol

household detergents

3 percent peroxide

We know that family members living with individuals who have the virus do not become infected except through sexual intercourse, or by blood from the infected person entering the bloodstream of another person.

Study after study shows that there is *no evidence whatsoever* of transmission of the virus by regular close contact, even though individuals shared food, towels, cups, razors, and even toothbrushes. Nor is there evidence of its being spread by mosquitoes or other insects, although researchers have transmitted the virus to mosquitoes by feeding them infected blood. Even in areas that are heavily infested with mosquitoes, only those people who are sexually active or who abuse IV drugs are infected with HIV.

Can AIDS Be Spread by Kissing?

On rare occasions the HIV virus has been found in the saliva of AIDS patients. In a study of fifty people with fully developed AIDS, the virus was found in only one

---

9. "A freshly prepared solution of sodium hypochlorite (household bleach) is an inexpensive and very effective germicide. Concentrations ranging from a 1:10 dilution of household bleach to a 1:100 dilution are effective, depending on the amount of organic material (e.g., blood, mucus, etc.) present on the surface to be cleaned and disinfected." *Morbidity and Mortality Weekly Report*, Centers for Disease Control, November 15, 1985.

saliva sample. There are no cases in which HIV is suspected of being transmitted by ordinary on-the-lips dry kissing.

On the other hand, deep, erotic kissing, or "French kissing" may be risky, and is not recommended, because of the exposure to large amounts of saliva.[10]

Dr. Anthony Fauci, of the National Institute of Allergy and Infectious Diseases, observes, "In order to be extra safe, health officials have to presume that it is possible to transmit the virus by exchange of saliva in deep kissing."

Inflamed gums and open sores or cavities in the mouth of the uninfected person would increase the risk of transmission.

HIV in Semen and Blood

HIV is transmitted from one person to another in blood and semen. These are the two primary body fluids with the highest concentration of cells. In an infected person, they would have the highest concentration of cells containing the HIV virus.

It may also be possible that HIV can be transmitted through vaginal secretions, although the virus seems to be less concentrated in vaginal secretions than in semen.

Semen contains sperm cells and, among other materials, white blood cells. Because the virus is carried in

---

10. While saliva by itself could not contain the virus, saliva could be contaminated by small amounts of infected blood that may come from bleeding gums or other damage to the lining of the mouth, throat, or tongue which would cause bleeding.

sperm and the white blood T-lymphocytes, the semen of an infected male can infect another person when it enters the vagina, anus, or possibly, the mouth.

There have been cases in which a woman with HIV infected her male sex partner. Researchers speculate that infected white T-lymphocytes in a woman's vaginal secretions, menstrual flow, discharge, or reproductive-tract infection could come into direct contact with the penis and be absorbed through the urethra, the duct in the male penis. The virus could also be absorbed through breaks in the urethra or the skin of the penis.

The Risks of Anal Intercourse

Anal intercourse—insertion of the penis into the rectum—is practiced by both homosexuals and heterosexuals.

Many studies have shown that when semen is released, the receptive partner in anal intercourse is at great risk of HIV infection.

The lining of the rectum is thin and easily irritated. There is more chance for tissue to be torn, causing bleeding and allowing the virus to spread through the cuts into the bloodstream.[11] In addition, the lining of the rectum is very absorbent. This is the reason doctors often choose to prescribe medications that can be given rectally. Because the rectal lining appears as if it has hundreds of microscopic hills and valleys, there is much more of that very absorbent surface exposed to the virus.

---

11. Consider how easy it is to break the skin and produce small amounts of blood when using toilet tissue after a bowel movement.

Studies also show that cells in the rectum and colon can become infected in anal intercourse.

The insertive partner in anal intercourse is also at risk. Three to 4 percent of HIV infections have taken place in men who always served as the insertive partner.

Oral Sex

Remember that the virus is found in both semen and vaginal secretions.

The risk of infection from oral sex increases if there are cuts in the mouth or on the gums or if semen is taken into the mouth. For these reasons, many researchers advise against oral sex unless you are absolutely sure that a person is not infected.

The Number of Sexual Partners

The risk of infection increases with the number of sexual partners a person has—male or female—because of greatly increased chances of being exposed to an infected partner.

Intravenous Drug Users

Drug abusers who inject drugs into their veins have high rates of infection by the AIDS virus. According to the Centers for Disease Control, users of intravenous drugs make up 25 percent of AIDS cases throughout the country. In some areas, IV drug abuse has become the most common way to become infected.

The AIDS virus is carried in contaminated blood left in the needle, syringe, or other drug-related implements. It is not uncommon for a single needle to be shared by as many as a dozen people. After each use, the needle is "cleaned" by such methods as licking it off, wiping it between the toes, or washing it in a toilet bowl. The virus is injected into the next person by reusing these dirty syringes and needles. Even the smallest amount of infected blood left in a used needle or syringe can contain the live AIDS virus, to be passed on to the veins of the next user.

Mother Can Infect the Unborn

A woman infected with HIV who becomes pregnant is putting herself and her unborn baby at great risk. She increases her own chance of developing ARC or AIDS, because pregnancy lowers her immunity and makes her more vulnerable to various infections. She can pass the virus on to her child primarily in the womb, and also during the birth or possibly through breast-feeding. An infected mother can transmit the disease even if she has no symptoms of AIDS.

While more studies are needed to better define that rate of transmission to infants, according to one study reported by the Centers for Disease Control, as many as 65 percent of the babies of HIV-infected mothers were born infected with the virus.

Most of the infected babies will eventually develop the disease and die.

Fully developed AIDS in infants is an unusually severe and fatal form of the disease.

Information Isn't Enough

Now you have the basic information about AIDS. But information doesn't protect you and your family. You have to *do something* with that information. It has to be applied to the kinds of practical questions about AIDS that are still unanswered. And that information has to move you to say no to the kinds of behavior that threaten your life and the lives of your family members.

Before we move on to the questions teens ask about AIDS, let's take a look at some surprising statistics on the sexual activity of "somebody's else's kids."

3

How Sexually Active Are Our Teenagers?

Mom was emptying the pockets of David's jeans, getting ready to do a load of clothes.

There was a note about homework. He was always forgetting that. Half a toothpick. A stub from the movies. And no money—as usual.

In the other pocket was a dirty handkerchief and a . . . a condom?

Her first response was shock. She turned the foil package over and over between her fingers. Then slowly, images began to fill her mind: David as a very little boy, David on his first day in school, David in Little League. . . .

She was almost overcome with a feeling of sadness. She had held on to the images of her *little boy*. Now, in her hands was the evidence that her "little boy" was gone forever.

"Or maybe he was just curious," she thought out loud. "There's all this talk on television. That must be it. . . ."

In her mind she saw David when he had pitched the winning game in the city championship last year. *A clean-looking boy*, she thought. And held on to that image, as she threw the foil packet in the wastebasket.

Not my David. She knew it couldn't be. "Not my David." She said it out loud this time as she put the jeans in the washer.

All across the country parents, like David's mom, are seeing glimpses of their teenagers' developing sexual interest—and like David's mom, many of us are finding it hard to believe.

We hear the reports of a million teenage pregnancies each year. But those things always seem to be happening somewhere else. "Not our kids," we are quick to point out.

It Has to Be Somebody's Kids

Sometimes just talking to teenagers at all can be difficult, let alone talking about sex—and now AIDS. We know we have to do it, but most of us will do it *when it's absolutely necessary.*

Before we talk about what to say, we need to look at just how necessary this heart-to-heart talk really is.

The percentages of our young people who are sexually active vary a little from survey to survey. Yet the surveys are consistent in saying the following:

- Sexual intercourse is not uncommon among children as young as twelve years old.

- By the time young people reach the age of seventeen, more than half of them have had sexual intercourse.

- By the time young people reach college age, three out of every four are sexually active.

Here's the way a typical mid-American teenager sees it: "If a guy and a girl date for more than a few weeks, everybody assumes they're making it in bed."

Blunt. But that's the world of today's teens. A world where sex is all around them.

What the Studies Tell Us

Researchers at Michigan State University[1] found that a large number of ninth- and tenth-grade girls watch between one and two hours of soap operas every day after school. And on the programs they watch, sexual intercourse between unmarried partners is shown or discussed an average of 1.56 times an hour.

In the evening, a larger number of ninth- and tenth-grade girls—and boys—watch three to four hours of television. On prime-time evening shows researchers recorded that, on the average, acts of unmarried intercourse were shown or discussed once an hour.

They also found that 60 to 70 percent of ninth- and tenth-graders saw the top five R-rated films. And here they saw sexual intercourse between unmarried partners an average of eight times per film. In the most sexually graphic films, sex occurred as much as fifteen times.

In that kind of world, is it any wonder that premarital sex seems okay to kids?

In a landmark study, psychiatrist Robert Coles and journalist Geoffrey Stokes surveyed teenage attitudes about sexual intercourse between teens who were

---

1. From a study by Dr. Bradley S. Greenburg, Michigan State University, Department of Telecommunications, August 1986.

1) strangers, 2) friends/dating, 3) going with each other, 4) in love, and 5) planning marriage.[2]

After months of carefully cross-checking all the data they had gathered, they made this observation:

> No matter where teens live, no matter what their race, family income, educational plans, grades, or religion, about 41% of them believe that love makes it permissible for a girl to have sexual intercourse when the couples are going steady. The impact of love is even more dramatic among girls than boys. Only 14% of all girls (including 13- and 14-year-olds, about 95% of whom disapprove) think it's okay for a girl going steady to have intercourse; but if the girl is "in love," more than 35% approve, including more than half the 17- and 18-year-olds.
>
> Yet the "in love" standard is extremely encompassing. Even at the age of 13, more than half of all teens (53% of boys, 52% of girls) say they have been in love, and the percentages finally rise to include 85% of 18-year-old boys and 83% of 17-year-old girls.

Then in summary, Geoffrey Stokes offered this thoughtful analysis of teens "in love":

> We have to remember what the survey showed about teens' conservatism. Teens do want their

---

2. Robert Coles and Geoffrey Stokes, *Sex and the American Teenager* (New York: Harper & Row Publishers, 1985).

59

friends to think well of them, and most do want to be "good." That combination can make the generous standard of love a flag of convenience. In the absence of notions like commitment and responsibility, horniness can look an awful lot like "love."

In any case, the attempt to form standards is different from living up to them, and among teens who've had sexual intercourse, two-thirds do not plan to marry their most recent sexual partner, a third say they did not love him or her, and a quarter say they weren't even girlfriend or boyfriend.

The research of Coles and Stokes also shows that most teens who have had intercourse once continue to be sexually active.

What Does It Mean to Be "Sexually Active"?

The information on the next few pages will surprise—and perhaps even shock—some parents. Others will have their suspicions confirmed. Except where noted, the statistics have been drawn from the study of Coles and Stokes, *Sex and the American Teenager,* and compared with other studies. There are no value judgments, no arguments about the pros and cons of a particular activity. My purpose has simply been to state, as clearly as possible, teenage participation in each activity.

As I ask you to take a look with me at the world of teenage sex, I need to confess that some of the things I found surprised me and—in the stark reality of AIDS—gave me great concern.

Masturbation

At least half of all boys and a quarter of all girls masturbate by age fifteen. This figure probably rises to about 85 percent for males and 60 percent for females by age twenty.[3] On the average, teens who masturbate start before they reach age twelve. Masturbation, or sexual self-gratification, is often accompanied by a fantasy drawn in some way from the young person's experience.

There is no danger of AIDS infection from sexual self-gratification.

Kissing

No one has ever counted the number of teens who kiss—or has ever needed to. The activity, it seems, is almost universal.

There is no danger of infection from lips-to-lips dry kissing. Because the virus has been found in saliva,[4] even though no case of infection has been traced solely to saliva, there is some risk in deep or French kissing—which does seem to be a frequent practice of teens. Again, no statistic on frequency could be found.

Touching Genitals

In the survey boys were asked, "Have you ever played with a girl's genitals with your hands?" Girls were asked if a boy had ever touched their genitals.

---

3. Catherine S. Chilman, *Adolescent Sexuality in a Changing American Society* (New York: John Wiley & Sons, 1983).
4. See chapter 4, Question 25, for a more detailed description of this risk.

Twenty-three percent of thirteen-year-old boys said they had touched a girl's genitals with their hands. At age fourteen and up the number jumped to 50 percent, climbed to 56 percent at age seventeen, and 61 percent at age eighteen.

At age thirteen, 18 percent of girls said that a boy had touched their genitals with his hands. The numbers do not climb significantly until age fifteen (37 percent), age sixteen (46 percent), age seventeen (61 percent), and age eighteen (60 percent).

When the question was asked about boys' genitals, 40 percent of the girls surveyed had touched a boy's penis.

There is some danger of contracting AIDS from vaginal secretions. If there were a cut or other break in the skin of the hands of the male, there is a slight chance that the virus from vaginal secretions of an infected female could enter the male's body.

It has been clearly established that the semen of an infected male does carry the AIDS virus. Again, there is a slight chance that, if the male is infected with the virus and is brought to a climax, semen containing the virus could enter the female's body through a break in the skin of the hands.

Same-Sex Experimentation

During the early teen years, same-sex experimentation is not uncommon. This can range, among boys, from comparing penis size to watching another masturbate, to mutual masturbation, to anal sex.

It appears that homosexual contacts are most common before age 15 and that the incidence is nigher for boys than girls. Sex play consisting of exhibitionism [exposure of the sexual organs], voyeurism [observing the sexual organs or sex acts of others] and mutual masturbation occurs fairly frequently in groups of boys between the ages of 8 and 13.[5]

Experimentation and same-sex play does not mean that the person has chosen or will choose a homosexual life-style. Because of fears of being labeled a homosexual, accurate figures on homosexual activity among teens are very difficult to establish. However, 5 percent of the teens surveyed by Coles and Stokes indicated that they had participated in some form of homosexual activity.

There is the same very slight risk of HIV infection in mutual masturbation as in genital play.

The high risk of anal sex is covered later under that subject.

Oral Sex

For many teens, oral sex comes before intercourse.

For some teenagers, oral sex is seen as part of foreplay, a less drastic step than intercourse in the progression of sexual commitment. On the other hand, many teenagers felt that oral stimulation of the genitals is a more intimate act

---

5. Chilman, *Adolescent Sexuality.*

than intercourse and, therefore, more likely to come after it. . . .[6]

According to teenagers surveyed for Coles and Stokes, girls and boys are almost exactly the same in feeling that oral sex is okay: with strangers (3 percent said it was okay), with friends who are dating (11 percent), when a couple is "going together" (23 percent), "in love" (36 percent), and if they are planning marriage (40 percent).

Oral sex is seen by girls as maintaining "technical virginity." In a study of Canadian university females, Edward Herald and Leslie Way found that "61 percent of the subjects had performed oral sex on their partners and 68 percent had experienced their partner performing oral sex on them." They also noted "the general increase in and acceptance of oral-genital sexual relations. . . . Whereas oral sex used to be viewed as a perverted type of behavior, it has now become a widely accepted practice."[7]

In mouth-to-genital sex, saliva is involved. The saliva of an AIDS-infected person has been found to contain the virus. However, there are no known cases of the virus being transmitted from saliva.[8]

Studies show that teenage girls tend to take the male's semen into their mouths and—in some cases—to swallow it. If the male is infected, this brings virus-carrying semen directly into the mouth, where it could infect the system through small cuts, bleeding gums, or cavities. The same

---

6. Aaron Hass, Ph.D., *Teenage Sexuality* (New York: Macmillan Publishing Company, 1979).

7. The *Journal of Sex Research*, Vol. 19, No. 4, November 1983.

8. *See* chapter 4, Question 25, for a more detailed description of this risk.

would be true of blood from a break in the skin of the penis.

We noted earlier that there is some evidence the virus can be carried in vaginal secretions. This would indicate that a male could take the virus into his mouth while performing oral sex on his partner.

Many AIDS experts advise against allowing semen to enter the mouth. When there is the possibility that the male may be infected, Dr. James Goedert of the National Cancer Institute recommends "mandatory condom use for all phases of every oral and vaginal contact."[9]

Anal Sex

While there are no figures on the number of teens who practice anal sex, there is evidence that many young people "try it." They hear it talked about among their friends. They're curious. At first, many girls are repulsed by the idea. But curiosity and a desire to please their mate sometimes take over.

Those who try it are placing themselves at serious risk. Receptive anal intercourse is the primary way the virus is transmitted among homosexuals. And for heterosexuals the best advice to women is "don't do it."[10]

Sex With a Stranger

Among teenage boys especially, casual sex (with girls) is not uncommon. In their research Coles and Stokes report:

9. "What Is Safe Sex?" *New England Journal of Medicine*, Vol. 316, No. 21, May 21, 1987.
10. See pages 52, 53 for the reasons anal intercourse is so risky.

Close to a third (31%) of nonvirgin boys have had sex with someone they "didn't really know," as opposed to about a fifth (22%) of the girls. In addition, boys were more than twice as likely (37%) to have first had intercourse with a stranger or friend, rather than a girlfriend or fiancée; only 17% of girls had done so.

Dr. Koop's advice on this type of sex is very clear:

Unless it is possible to know with *absolute certainty* that neither you nor your sexual partner is carrying the virus of AIDS, you must use protective behavior. *Absolute certainty* means not only that you and your partner have maintained a mutually faithful, monogamous sexual relationship, but it means that neither you nor your partner has used illegal intravenous drugs.[11]

Dr. Goedert of the National Cancer Institute observes that "in the majority of the population [who have not been tested for AIDS and found to be negative] each partner must be considered potentially at risk or contagious."[12]

The Surgeon General—and others—have also said very bluntly that when you have sex with someone you are really having sex with all the other person's sex part-

---

11. From the *Surgeon General's Report on AIDS*.
12. *New England Journal of Medicine*, Vol. 316, No. 21, May 21, 1987.

ners—and their partners' partners—for the last ten years (or for as long as the partner has been sexually active, if less than ten years).

Changing Sexual Partners

Most teenage sex takes place in some kind of relationship. But that relationship may be very temporary.

Almost one-fifth, or 19 percent, of boys, the Coles and Stokes survey showed, and one-tenth of girls, or 9 percent, said their most recent sexual relationship had endured a week or less. Only 14 percent of all the teenagers' sexual relationships had lasted more than a year.

The same survey found that about one-quarter, or 26 percent, of the nonvirgin boys and one-tenth, or 11 percent, of the girls have had more than one sexual relationship going on at the same time.

In his study of teenage sexuality, Dr. Aaron Hass found that at age fifteen to sixteen, 54 percent of boys and 85 percent of girls had intercourse with one to five partners. At age seventeen to eighteen, the figure for boys (with one to five partners) increased to 60 percent, while girls decreased slightly to 83 percent. At age fifteen to sixteen, 28 percent of the boys and 7 percent of the girls surveyed had intercourse with more than ten partners. At age seventeen to eighteen, the numbers of boys with more than ten partners dropped to 28 percent, while the figure for girls of the same age dropped to 5 percent.[13]

The Surgeon General says very plainly:

---

13. Hass, *Teenage Sexuality.*

The risk of infection increases according to the number of sexual partners one has, male or female. The more partners you have, the greater the risk of being infected with the virus.

In the next chapter, we will find out what this high-risk generation wants to know about AIDS.

4

101 Questions Kids Ask About AIDS

If an educational campaign is to change behavior that spreads HIV infection, its message must be as direct as possible. [We] must be willing to use whatever vernacular is required for that message to be understood. Admonitions to avoid "intimate body contact" and the "exchange of bodily fluid" convey at best only a vague message.

National Academy of Sciences[1]

There are certainly no "vague messages" in the questions kids ask about AIDS. The questions are blunt. Direct. Sometimes even crude. Kids generally don't use clinical words when they're talking about sex.

One Monday afternoon after school I sat in a junior high school auditorium watching kids come in to hear a doctor talk about AIDS. Each student passed a permission slip to the teacher at the door.

---

1. National Academy of Sciences, *Confronting AIDS* (Washington, D.C., National Academy Press, 1986).

Once inside the auditorium, some students hung around the back of the room looking for friends. Most came in groups of two or three. There was a lot of moving from seat to seat, a lot of nervous laughter as they waited for the talk to begin.

The doctor gave a teenage version of some of the material you read in chapter 2.

Finally, it was time for questions. Blank cards were distributed. Questions were written down and passed in. The questions those young teens asked are a part of this chapter.

From New York to San Francisco I talked with medical doctors and health educators to gather the questions they had been asked by kids. Some questions I heard over and over again, like the "Can I Get AIDS From . . ." Questions and those that dealt with sexual practice and protection. And sometimes a single troubled teen would ask a new question.

The questions in this chapter, then, are real. They reflect genuine fears and a high level of sexual awareness and activity. And, unfortunately, sometimes they reflect serious misinformation, the kind any youngster can pick up from the guy or gal who pretends to know "from experience."

I have tried to keep the answers as simple as possible. Each one has been carefully reviewed for medical accuracy. Remember that no answer to a simple question can give you the complete AIDS story. Along with each set of questions I suggest that you reread the basic information in chapter 1.

If you have further questions or want to know more about specific questions, be sure to talk with your physician. You may also call the National AIDS Hotline: 1-800-342-AIDS.

Some Basic Questions

1. What is AIDS?

AIDS means *acquired immune deficiency syndrome*. The body's natural immune system is destroyed by this disease. As a result it cannot protect itself against infections and cancers.

2. What causes AIDS?

AIDS is caused by a virus that scientists call HIV (human immunodeficiency virus).

3. How does a person get AIDS?

AIDS is spread through direct blood-to-blood or semen-to-blood contact.

The virus is passed from one person to another *chiefly* during sexual contact, through sharing dirty needles and syringes used to shoot illegal drugs, or through transmission of blood or blood products contaminated by the virus.[2] It can also be passed from an infected pregnant mother to her unborn child.

4. How did AIDS get started?

Some researchers believe that the virus first appeared in central Africa in the mid-1970s. Most

---

2. Since May 1985, all donated blood in the United States has been tested for HIV. *See* page 48 for a more detailed explanation.

people with AIDS in Africa are heterosexuals and are not drug abusers, and as many women as men are infected.

As to *how* it got started we have no proof, only rumors, and leading scientists from around the world have refuted each of the rumors.

5. Is AIDS in other countries?

Yes. AIDS cases have been reported in 132 countries. Around the world equal numbers of women and men are infected—and it is *primarily transmitted by heterosexuals.*

6. How many people have AIDS now?

In the United States it is estimated that between a million and a million and a half people are *infected* with the virus. There are thirty-five thousand cases of fully developed AIDS, and about twenty thousand of these people have died.

The World Health Organization estimates that, worldwide, between five and ten million people may now be infected with the virus. Over fifty thousand cases of fully developed AIDS have been reported. WHO experts estimate that the *actual* number of cases is in excess of one hundred thousand worldwide.

7. How many will get it in the future?

Researchers estimate that by 1991, ten years after the disease was first identified, there will be 270,000 reported cases of fully developed AIDS in the United States, and 179,000 of these victims will have died.

8. Why did so many homosexual males in this country catch it first?

Because some homosexuals have many sex partners in a single night or a weekend, a few men with AIDS infected large numbers of gay men in a short time.

9. Why is AIDS more common for homosexuals?

It is only more common for homosexuals *in the United States.* In some other parts of the world as many women as men are infected.

Some homosexual men practice anal intercourse (in anal intercourse the penis is inserted into the rectum of a partner). The lining of the rectum is very absorbent and is easily torn, creating a high risk that semen infected with HIV will come into direct contact with the partner's blood. Since the beginning of the AIDS epidemic, there seems to have been a major reduction in this practice among gay men.

10. I'm not a homosexual. I can't get AIDS, can I?

Yes, you can! The AIDS virus can be transmitted in heterosexual intercourse with an infected person and in other kinds of sexual activity.

It can also be transmitted by sharing dirty IV needles and syringes that contain small amounts of infected blood, and by receiving transfusions of contaminated blood.

AIDS is not contracted because of what you *are*, but because of what you *do*.

11. Why do young people have a greater risk of getting AIDS?

Because many sexually active young people

a. change partners frequently,
b. engage in sex more frequently, and
c. may also be involved in IV drug abuse.

Young people need to realize that *whenever you have sex with someone, you are also having sex with everyone else your partner has had sex with.*

Here is a very painful fact: Twenty-one percent of fully developed AIDS cases reported to the Centers for Disease Control are in the twenty- to twenty-nine-year age group. Because it can take five years or more for symptoms to develop, this means that these people could have been infected between the ages of fifteen and twenty-four.

12. Does a person have to have symptoms of AIDS to give the virus to someone else?

No. Most people with the virus have no symptoms and do not know they are infected. Any person who is infected with the virus, whether or not they have any AIDS symptoms, can infect another person if there is direct semen-to-blood or blood-to-blood contact.

The infected person will *always* have the virus in his or her system.

13. Does everyone who is infected with the AIDS virus get fully developed AIDS?

No. Ten to 30 percent of those who are infected with the virus will have fully developed AIDS within five years.

Dr. Anthony Fauci, a leading AIDS researcher, says that it could be as long as twelve to fifteen years before AIDS symptoms show up.

14. Does everybody who gets AIDS die?

Yes. More than half the people who contracted AIDS have already died, and the rest probably will.

More than 50 percent of those with fully developed AIDS die within the first year.

Almost 95 percent die within two years.

15. Why do IV drug abusers get AIDS?

IV drug abusers often get together to share needles and other drug equipment. Before a needle is passed from one user to the next it is often licked off or wiped between the toes. Because of this, small amounts of blood from an infected person can be left in the dirty needle or syringe. It can then be injected directly into the bloodstream of the next drug abuser . . . and the next. . . .

16. How do children get AIDS?

Most children with fully developed AIDS contracted the virus from the blood of their infected mothers in the womb or during birth. A few received transfusions of contaminated blood or blood products.

17. Can a pregnant woman pass the AIDS virus on to her baby?

Yes. As many as 65 percent of infected mothers pass the virus on to their babies.

There is no way to know in advance if a baby will be infected. Twins were born to an infected mother; one was born with the virus and the other was not.

A woman who has the AIDS virus should not have children.

18. How would I know if I had AIDS?

If you have been involved in an activity in which you might have become infected, the only way to find out whether you do or do not have the AIDS virus in your system is to have an AIDS blood test. (*See* Questions 76 through 88.)

Remember that you can have the virus in your system for a long time before developing any symptoms.

19. What are some of the symptoms of AIDS?

When a person has fully developed AIDS, more and more T-lymphocytes are being destroyed until the body's immune system cannot protect itself against germs and cancers that would normally not be able to gain a foothold. These are called "opportunistic diseases." They use the body's lowered resistance as an opportunity to infect and destroy the body.

Some symptoms of fully developed AIDS and these opportunistic infections may include a persistent cough and fever with shortness of breath or difficult breathing. These may be the symptoms of Pneumocystis carinii pneumonia (new-mo-SIS-tis kar-IN-e-eye noo-MOAN-e-uh). While the Pneumocystis carinii parasite is in the system of most humans, it causes no trouble or symptoms. However, when the body's immune system is destroyed, the parasite causes this very destructive type of pneumonia. This is what kills a large number of people with AIDS.

Infected individuals may also develop certain types of cancers such as Kaposi's sarcoma (KAP-oh-sees sar-COMB-uh). This cancer produces purplish blotches and bumps on or under the skin, inside the mouth, eyelids, nose, and rectum. It is one of the visible and often disfiguring signs of fully developed AIDS.

20. I heard some people talk about ARC. What is that?

ARC means AIDS-Related Complex. It is a name used to describe symptoms of HIV infection which are not as severe as the disease we call fully developed AIDS. Some individuals with ARC die without having fully developed AIDS. Up to now about 20 to 30 percent of the people with ARC have developed the diseases that are fatal to people with fully developed AIDS. This figure may change as we have more experience with the virus.

The signs and symptoms of ARC are listed on pages 45, 46.

21. Can a person get infected more than once?

Once is enough. Once is forever. There is no cure for AIDS.

22. Is it easier for people who live in a big city to get AIDS?

No. Sexual activity is not limited to big cities. AIDS cases have now been reported in every part of the United States. There are also cases in smaller cities, towns, and rural areas.

You don't contract the virus because of where you *live*. You contract it because of what you *do*.

23. Does smoking break down the ability to fight off the virus?

There is no evidence that this is true. However, smokers are subject to respiratory infections. If a smoker gets ARC or fully developed AIDS, he/she may have more serious complications.

"Can I Get AIDS From . . . ?" Questions

24. Can I get AIDS from sharing a soda?

No. To get the virus, the blood or semen of an infected person must come in direct contact with the blood of another person.

25. Can I get AIDS from kissing?

In a survey of teens, 57 percent thought you could contract AIDS by kissing a person with AIDS. The truth is that dry lip-to-lip kissing appears safe. There is *absolutely no record* of the virus being transmitted this way.

Deep or French kissing *may* be dangerous since saliva is exchanged. While saliva *by itself* could not contain the virus, saliva *could* be contaminated by small amounts of infected blood from pyorrhea (pie-oh-REE-ah), bleeding gums, sore throat, and ulcers, cuts, and scrapes in the mouth. The virus has been found in saliva which contained small amounts of blood, which could come in contact with cuts or breaks in the surface of the gums and the inside of the mouth of the partner.

26. Can I get AIDS from tears?

No. While the virus has been found in tears, experts estimate that you would have to "main-line"—inject directly into the vein—about two gallons of tears from an infected person to be infected by the virus.

The Centers for Disease Control report that "there is no evidence to date that [HIV] has been transmitted through contact with the tears of infected individuals."[3]

27. Can I get AIDS from mosquitoes?

There is no record that mosquitoes, other insects, or rodents can spread the disease to humans, although researchers have transmitted the virus to mosquitoes by feeding them infected blood.

28. Can I get AIDS from drinking from the same glass or eating from the same dishes as someone infected with the virus?

No. The virus is killed by normal dish washing. There has never been a case of AIDS reported to be caused by sharing glasses, dishes, or eating utensils.

29. Can I get AIDS from the telephone?

No.

30. Can I get AIDS from sharing makeup?

No. You have to have blood-to-blood or semen-to-blood contact with an infected person to be infected with the virus.

---

3. *Morbidity and Mortality Weekly Report,* Centers for Disease Control, August 30, 1985.

31. Can I get AIDS from touching someone who has it?

No. AIDS is not spread by casual day-to-day contact. Remember . . . there has to be blood-to-blood or semen-to-blood contact.

32. Can I get AIDS from shaking hands or hugging?

Lots of young people think this is true, but the answer is NO.

33. Can I get AIDS just by going to school with someone who has the virus or fully developed AIDS?

No, unless you have sexual contact with that person, or share an IV needle.

(For Public Health Service Guidelines on Education and Foster Care of Children Infected With HIV, see Appendix B.)

34. I know someone who is gay. Can I get AIDS from being around him?

No. Remember that AIDS is not a gay (homosexual) disease. *All gay people are not infected with the AIDS virus.*

And even if the person you know *is* infected, there is no danger of infection from casual, friendly contact. You would be at risk only if you had sexual contact with your infected friend, or if he or she passed you an IV needle that had already been used.

35. If somebody's blood gets on me, in an accident, for example, could I get AIDS?

No, unless that person is infected with the virus, and you have broken skin (so that there is the possibility of blood-to-blood contact). If your skin has been broken by a needle, a cut or laceration, an abrasion (such as a skinned knee), a maceration (where the skin is rubbed until it begins to be worn down or away, as with a pressure sore), or you have dermatitis or any other form of damage to the skin, your skin should immediately be washed with any of the disinfectants listed on page 50.

36. Can I get AIDS from taking a bath in a bathtub that has been used by someone with AIDS?

No. The virus cannot be contracted by touching something that has been used by a person with fully developed AIDS.

37. Is it possible to get AIDS from someone swimming in a pool?

No. If the virus were in the water, it would be killed by the chlorine in the pool.

38. Can I get AIDS from a toilet seat?

Absolutely not.

39. Can I get AIDS from a water fountain?

No. The virus is not transmitted by water or by touching anything used by a person with AIDS.

40. Can I get AIDS if someone coughs or sneezes in my direction?

No. The virus cannot be transmitted through the air.

41. Can I get AIDS if somebody bites me?

The virus has been found in saliva which has picked up the virus from blood from the mouth, so it *is* possible. However, there are no AIDS cases suspected of being caused by a bite.

42. Can I get AIDS by *giving* blood?

No. All blood banks use sterile equipment to draw blood. Needles are thrown away after being used *only once.*

There is *no possibility* of the virus being spread by giving blood—though 60 percent of surveyed teens thought they could be infected by giving blood.

43. Are blood transfusions safe?

Prior to early 1985 some people did contract the virus through receiving blood and blood products, but since then all donated blood in the United States has been screened for antibodies to the virus. After the test, all blood which has antibodies to HIV is destroyed. As a result, a hospital's supply of blood and blood products (such as those used in treating hepatitis and hemophilia) is now as safe as is humanly possible.

As an extra safety measure, doctors are more cautious in ordering blood transfusions.

Questions About Sexual Practices

> The number of teens who are "not worried" about contracting AIDS is on the increase. In 1986, 54 percent indicated they were "not worried," compared to 34 percent in 1985.[4]

44. Is one type of sex riskier than another?

In anal intercourse, when the insertive partner is infected with the AIDS virus, the receptive partner faces a very high risk. (See pages 52, 53 for a more detailed explanation.)

There is also a significant risk in heterosexual intercourse when both partners have not maintained an absolutely faithful sexual relationship to each other for the last ten years.

Having a number of sex partners increases the risk of contracting AIDS.

There is some risk of contracting AIDS from any sexual activity that involves the possibility of direct semen-to-blood, blood-to-semen, or blood-to-blood contact.

(See pages 47–54 for more details on how AIDS is transmitted.)

---

4. Lee Strunin, Ph.D., and Ralph Hingson, Sc.D., "Acquired Immunodeficiency Syndrome and Adolescents: Knowledge, Beliefs, Attitudes and Behaviors," *Pediatrics*, Vol. 79, No. 5, May 1987.

45. Can women transmit AIDS?

Yes. The HIV virus has been found in vaginal fluid, particularly when it is mixed with menstrual blood.

46. Do prostitutes spread AIDS?

Yes. Prostitutes are often infected with the virus because they have a large number of sex partners, and many prostitutes are IV drug abusers.

Like any other person infected with the virus, prostitutes are able to infect others.

Here is the important thing to remember: *Anyone who is sexually involved with an unknown partner increases the risk of contracting AIDS.*

47. Isn't is true that homosexuals who have only one or two partners won't get AIDS?

To be in a sexual realtionship with a *single partner* in which each has been *totally faithful* to the other for ten years or more, and in which neither has shared dirty IV needles, is to eliminate the risk of contracting AIDS.

But whether you are a homosexual or a heterosexual, when you have more than one sex partner, it becomes very difficult to guarantee that a partner is not infected with the virus.

48. Why is it easier to get AIDS through anal intercourse?

The lining of the rectum is thin and can easily be torn in anal intercourse. This makes it easier for the virus to be passed on from semen to the blood through torn tissue. (*See* pages 52, 53 for a more complete explanation.)

49. Is it possible that I won't get AIDS if I have sex with someone who has it?

Yes. It is *possible*, if a condom is put on before there is any genital contact, it is worn from the beginning to the end of sex, it does not break, no semen is spilled when the condom is removed, there is no deep or French kissing, and no oral sex. But make no mistake, *you are playing with fire.* In this situation, the only way to be absolutely sure you are not going to be infected with HIV (the AIDS virus) is to *avoid oral, anal, or vaginal intercourse.*

50. I just sleep with my friends, and they're clean. I'm not in danger of contracting AIDS, am I?

First of all, how do you know they're "clean"? Have you talked about it in detail, or are you just asssuming they're "clean"? If you sleep with a number of people, isn't it reasonable to assume that they do, too? And can you be sure that *all of their partners* are not infected—or that there isn't an IV drug abuser among them?

The big problem is that you sleep with "friends"— plural. And having more than one sex partner puts you at much greater risk.

51. I'm only thirteen. I'm too young to get AIDS, aren't I?

It isn't your age, it's your *activity* that could get you infected. If you are involved in oral sex, anal or vaginal intercourse, you can be infected by the AIDS virus, regardless of how old you are.

52. If I'm careful about sex, that's enough, isn't it?

In one survey, 25 percent of kids between sixteen and nineteen said that because of AIDS, they had decided to be "careful."

What does it mean to be "careful"? You've got to be more specific than that. Being "careful" is not adequate protection.

You must decide to abstain from sex, use a condom from start to finish, or be absolutely sure that your partner has not engaged in activity which could have caused infection.

53. If I'm not infected and I have sex with someone who isn't infected, can I still get AIDS?

No. The infection is not caused by the fact that you had intercourse. The virus is passed on by an infected person.

But you need to be *absolutely sure* that a sex partner has not been infected. Remember that having sex with someone is really having sex with every other person they've had intercourse with, and all the sex partners of those people, for the last ten years (or as long as they've been sexually active, if that is less than ten years).

54. Is there a greater chance of a woman getting AIDS from a man than a man getting AIDS from a woman?

Yes. The number of cases in which women have been infected with the virus by men is increasing.

It is less likely that the virus will spread from a woman to a man on a single exposure.

55. Does the birth control pill block out AIDS?

No. It provides no protection whatsoever from AIDS.

In a survey of teens, 22 percent did not know that the AIDS virus is transmitted by semen, and 29 percent did not know that it can be transmitted by vaginal fluids.

---

56. Can I get AIDS from masturbation?

No. In masturbation, or self-gratification, there is no contact with the blood or semen of any other person.

57. Can I get AIDS from mutual masturbation?

The risk is not high, but it *could* happen if infected semen or blood were to come in contact with a break in the skin.

58. Can I get AIDS from "making out"?

It all depends on what *you* mean by "making out." This term means different things to different people.

As long as "making out" doesn't mean oral, anal, or vaginal intercourse, or the possibility of semen-to-blood or blood-to-blood contact (where open cuts could come in contact with infected semen or blood), there is no danger of contracting AIDS.

59. Can I get AIDS from touching someone else's genitals?

There is *very little risk.*

In touching a female's genitals, you could get vaginal fluid on your hands where it could come into contact with a cut or abrasion. During menstruation, perhaps because of the flow of blood, the virus has been found in vaginal fluid.

60. Can I get AIDS from oral sex?

The risk of infection from oral sex is not clear. However, there could be a risk if there are cuts, scrapes, ulcers, or bleeding gums in the mouth or if semen is taken into the mouth. Many researchers advise against oral sex unless you can be absolutely sure that your partner is not infected. Of course, to be absolutely safe, the best answer is abstinence.

61. Can I get AIDS from swallowing semen?

Yes, if the person whose semen you take into your mouth is infected with the AIDS virus. It's not the swallowing that is the problem, but the possibility of taking infected semen into your mouth. (See the answer to Question 60.)

62. Can Lesbians get AIDS?

It is extremely unlikely because their sexual practices would make blood-to-blood or vaginal fluid-to-blood contact almost impossible. They could, how-ever, contract AIDS through dirty IV needles or contaminated blood, just like anyone else.

63. Am I more likely to get AIDS if I have a number of sex partners?

Yes. The number of partners increases the risk. It's simple—you are more likely to have sex with some-one who is infected with the virus.

64. If my clitoris were touched by a guy's penis, just on the outside, could I get AIDS?

Clear preseminal fluid, which serves as a natural lubricant, can be released from the penis before the male climaxes. In this situation, that small amount of fluid would have to be infected, and you would have to be close enough for that semen to reach your vagina, or any other cut or abrasion on your body.

You would also be wise to consider whether it is likely you would stop with this limited sexual con-tact.

65. Can I get AIDS if he withdraws in time?

Yes. If there is a possibility that he is infected, this can't be considered a safe practice. Infected semen can be released from the penis before he climaxes.

And in the rush of powerful emotions, you may not be able to be sure that his penis *has* been withdrawn.

66. Could I get AIDS from being molested?

Yes, if the molester is infected with the virus and any sex act takes place which involves semen-to-blood contact.

67. My boyfriend says he's safe because he hasn't had sex with anyone else. Can I believe him?

You may want very much to believe him—for lots of reasons. But unless you can be *absolutely sure* that he has not had sex with anyone else in the last ten years (or as long as he has been sexually active), your answer should be no—unless he is willing to use a condom. For teenagers, the safest solution is to say no.

68. So many times doctors say, "You could get AIDS this way or that." Don't we know for sure?

While we have learned a lot about AIDS since it was first identified in 1981, there is still a great deal we do not know.

The more we learn about the virus, the more we can speak with assurance. But sex partners often engage in a number of different sexual activities, and it is difficult to know which activity was the one in which the virus was transmitted. Until we can know for sure that the virus absolutely cannot be contracted in one particular kind of sexual activity, we can only say things such as, "There is no record of the virus being transmitted this way," or, "As far as we know now. . . ."

We can know without any doubt whatsoever that AIDS *is* transmitted by sexual contact, IV drug abuse with shared dirty needles, receiving transfusions of contaminated blood, and from a pregnant mother to her unborn or newborn child.

We also know that high-risk sexual activities are receptive anal sex, sharing IV drug needles and syringes, having sex with someone you are not *absolutely sure* is free of the virus, or changing sexual partners frequently.

Questions About Condoms

69. What is a condom?

People often call them "rubbers." A condom is a thin, balloonlike latex cover placed over the erect penis before intercourse and carefully removed after withdrawal from the vagina. Some so-called natural condoms are made from the intestinal tissue of lambs. (See pages 147–149 for more details on condoms and their use.)

70. Are condoms safe?

No condom is 100 percent safe. They have been known to break or come off during use. Condoms have only been tested in laboratories, not in actual use.

According to the U.S. Food and Drug Administration, one out of every five batches of condoms tested in laboratories by the government in mid-1987 failed to meet minimum standards for leakage. They only provide *safer sex* when they are used properly and worn from the beginning to the end of intercourse, and are removed carefully so that no semen is spilled.

71. Can the AIDS virus pass through a condom?

Many health experts are unwilling to say yes or no. "We cannot tell people how much protection condoms give," says Dr. Malcolm Potts, one of the inventors of prophylactics lubricated with spermicide. So-called lambskin condoms contain pores that could allow the tiny HIV virus to escape. The FDA has requested that manufacturers of natural condoms discontinue use of any claims that the products are capable of preventing transmission of any sexually transmitted disease.

72. For a condom to work, do I have to use it in a special way?

Yes. Unless there is a reservoir tip, you must leave space at the tip, it must be put on before any insertion of the penis, and be carefully removed and disposed of after final withdrawal of the penis. (See pages 147, 148 for specific instructions on proper use of a condom.)

73. If I keep a condom in my wallet for a few days, will it still be good?

The more chance there is for a condom to dry out, the more risk there is that it will crack or break.

74. If a condom is washed out, can it be used again?

Absolutely not. Condoms are designed for *one-time use only*.

75. Is a diaphragm as good a protection against AIDS as a condom?

No. A diaphragm only protects the woman's cervix. Without the male using a condom, infected sperm will still contact the walls of the vagina, creating a risk of infection.

Questions About AIDS Testing

76. What is the AIDS test?

The HIV virus causes antibodies to be developed in the bloodstream. A simple blood test can detect those antibodies. *It does not test for the virus directly.* If the test results are positive (HIV antibodies are found in the blood), a second—and different—test is performed.

If the second test also shows a positive result, the person has been infected with the virus.

If the test is negative, this usually means that the person has *not* been infected. However, the test will not show infections within the past six to twelve weeks. Persons who have practiced high-risk behaviors during the past six to twelve weeks need to maintain several months of abstinence or "safe sex," then be tested again.

77. Is the test accurate?

It is almost 100 percent accurate. The first test could give a false positive report once or twice in one hundred tests. The possibility of error is virtually eliminated by the second test.

78. How long does it take for antibodies to develop?

In most cases, antibodies to the virus will develop within six to twelve weeks after infection.

79. Who should take the AIDS test?

You should take the test if you have had sex with a person you now know has AIDS, uses IV drugs, has hemophilia, or is an active homosexual or bisexual. You should also be tested if you received blood or blood products between 1978 and April 1985—at which point testing began on all donated blood in the United States, or if a medical doctor suspects that your symptoms may be AIDS-related.

80. Is the test dangerous?

No. A small amount of blood is drawn from the arm, and a new, clean needle is used each time.

81. Does a positive test mean I will get fully developed AIDS?

Most people with a positive test are totally without symptoms of AIDS. At the present, about 30 to 40 percent will develop minor symptoms (ARC), and about 10 to 30 percent will eventually have fully developed AIDS.

It appears that in the future many, if not most, of the people with a positive test will develop ARC. It is not known how many will have fully developed AIDS.

82. Does a positive test mean I can infect someone else?

Yes. In fact, *as soon as you are infected, you can infect someone else.*

If you have continued to have sex between the time you were infected and the time you were tested, you have most likely infected your sex partner(s).

A positive test means that you should now refrain from sex with anyone.

83. If I have a positive test, does that mean I can't get married?

There is no law that says you can't get married. But the person you want to marry needs to be told that you are infected and that sexual intercourse would place her or him at very great risk.

84. If a woman's test is positive, can she have a baby?

Any children born to a mother infected with the virus face a 50 percent chance of being born with AIDS.

85. Are AIDS tests really secret?

If the test is *anonymous*, as it is in many cities and states, your name is never asked for or recorded. Your test is identified only by a number, and the results will only be given to you in person.

If the test is described as *confidential*, you will be asked to give your name, but in most states the results are kept secret. In Arizona, Colorado, Florida, Idaho, Minnesota, Montana, South Carolina, Wisconsin, and an increasing number of states, positive test results have to be reported to the state health department.

86. How much does the test cost?

The test is offered free of charge in public health clinics. However, you will generally have to make an appointment, then wait several weeks after the test for the result. Your local public health office will give you the locations of testing clinics.

Some private labs are charging fifty to sixty dollars for the basic AIDS test—called an ELISA (e-LIE-za) test. The Western blot test is usually in the same price range.

Wherever you are tested, be sure that counseling is offered. Regardless of the results of the test, it is essential that you talk with a professional about the ways your sexual or IV drug activity should change in order to eliminate risk to yourself or others.

87. If my AIDS test is negative, does that mean I won't get AIDS?

A negative test *usually* means that you have not been infected. However, the test shows the presence (or absence) or antibodies to the virus, and it takes six to twelve weeks after infection for antibodies to develop.

If, within the time since the possible infection, the tested person has had additional sexual or IV drug activity which could have caused infection, a negative test does not guarantee that the person is free of infection.

Recently, a new blood test was developed that, because it directly indicates the presence of antigens to the AIDS virus, may provide earlier detection of the HIV virus.

A negative test does not mean that you are immune. It is no guarantee that you will not become infected as a result of sexual activity in the future.

88. When people have positive AIDS tests, are they honest about the results?

People who know they are infected, and who really care about a potential sexual partner, would want the person to know the risk they face. But that is not true in every case.

Because people with AIDS are often discriminated against in jobs and housing, those with positive test results will generally want to keep the information secret from the public.

More Questions on Protection and Treatment

89. By the time I get AIDS, won't there be a cure?

Wait a minute! That's *really* gambling—with your life and the lives of others.

You know that there is no cure available now. This is a fatal disease. Researchers predict that there may be a vaccine to protect against the virus by the end of the century. We are beginning to see drugs such as AZT, which can treat some of the diseases related to fully developed AIDS, but no researcher will predict when a cure will be available. If you were to be infected, you could exhibit symptoms of the fully developed disease *within months.*

We're dealing with a fatal disease that is transmitted through sexual activity. Unless you know that your sex partner, and every person he/she has had sex with for the last ten years (if they've been sexually active that long), is not infected, you are playing with fire.

90. Penicillin will cure AIDS, won't it?

No. Penicillin kills only certain *bacteria.* AIDS is caused by a *virus.* Penicillin has no effect on viruses. There is no drug now available that will cure AIDS, nor is there likely to be one for many years to come.

91. Would it help if I took lots of vitamins?

A healthy body can help fight off infection, but there is no evidence that vitamins can keep you from contracting the virus or developing ARC or fully developed AIDS.

92. Isn't there a vaccine to prevent AIDS?

No. Scientists are working very hard at this, but most of them believe that it will be at least the middle to late 1990s before a vaccine can be developed, tested, and made available to the public.

93. What is AZT?

Azidothymidine (a-ZY-do-THIGH-mah-deen) or AZT—now known as Retrovir®—prevents the AIDS virus from multiplying.

94. Does AZT cure AIDS?

No, but in a selected few patients with fully developed AIDS, AZT appears to prolong and improve their quality of life. Extensive research is under way to develop other drugs.

95. Can I destroy the AIDS virus by washing my hands often?

The virus is transmitted only by semen-to-blood and blood-to-blood contact. It is not transmitted by day-to-day casual contact. However, cleanliness is always wise if you help take care of a person who has *any* kind of infectious disease. The AIDS virus is destroyed by many methods, including the ones explained on page 50. Hot water, regular hand soap, and the friction of washing your hands will also destroy the virus.

96. When will there be other drugs for treating AIDS patients?

Experiments are being done with other drugs right now. Each is being very carefully tested. The Food and Drug Administration is doing everything possible to ensure that new drugs to treat AIDS patients are absolutely safe and are made available as soon as possible.

Final Questions

97. Is AIDS hereditary?

No.

98. Could a child born with the virus (but who never got the disease) pass it on to a child of his/her own later on?

Because we have known about AIDS for such a short time, there is no recorded case of this, but there is a possiblity that it could happen.

99. Can a person with the AIDS virus catch other diseases more easily?

Yes. Because the immune system is destroyed, other infections can take hold more easily.

100. Why aren't AIDS victims quarantined?

People with AIDS or those infected with the virus do not pass the virus on through casual contact. They pose no risk in day-to-day contact. A quarantine would serve no useful purpose, and it would be virtually impossible to quarantine the large numbers of people who are believed to be infected.

Quarantines have been used only with diseases that can be contracted by respiratory or casual contact such as tuberculosis, mumps, measles.

If we avoid the activities that cause infection, *we are all safe*. That is self-quarantine, and that is the only effective quarantine.

101. Can people with AIDS go to work? Shouldn't they be kept from working in places like restaurants, hospitals, barbershops?

AIDS victims can work as long as they are well enough. They should, of course, take precautions that no one comes into contact with their blood, without immediately providing disinfectant.

There is no risk of contracting AIDS through the air, or from water or food. No cases of AIDS have ever been reported as a result of casual contact.

For Public Health Service Guidelines on Preventing Transmission of Infection in the Workplace, see Appendix C.

PART 2

Getting the Message to Our Kids

So far, we've talked about the fact that many of today's teens risk contracting AIDS.

We've talked about AIDS and how it is—and isn't—transmitted. And we've looked at the questions teens ask about AIDS.

The Surgeon General has said that "parents . . . cannot disregard [the] responsibility to educate our young. The need is critical and the price of neglect is high. The lives of our young people depend on our fulfilling our responsibility."

The first step in taking that responsibility seriously is to know the facts about AIDS. We've been looking at those facts in chapters 1 through 4.

The following chapters can help prepare you to talk with your preteens and teens with knowledge, sensitivity, and patience.

5

"Please Understand Me"

"**Y**ou're not *listening* to me."

The teenager fought back tears. Hot tears of frustration.

Once the words were said . . . you could see her pulling away from the argument.

Then pain turned to fire. Frustration gave way to anger as she stormed down the hall to her bedroom.

"You *never* listen to me."

And the bedroom door slammed behind her.

You're left alone with a host of conflicting emotions:

"That was unfair. I *do* try to listen."

"Every time we talk . . . it seems to end up this way. . . ."

"*My* mother would never let me talk to her that way."

"We're growing apart, and I don't know why. I try to talk to her. . . . It's like she's a different person."

Sometimes this mother-daughter battle goes on for days. Other times it ends before long in the warmth of restoration.

"I love you, Mom. Sometimes I don't know what gets

into me. . . ." The little-girl-now-growing-up gives you a hug, and leans her head on your shoulder.

And you return the hug—grateful for the peace. Hoping this was the last battle, yet knowing it won't be. Knowing there is more pain, more confusion, more assertiveness, and much more growing ahead. You want it all to happen—because it must—yet you wish it could all be over, this time called adolescence.

"You don't listen to me." That's probably a teenager's most common complaint. And often unspoken, but just as real, is another: "Nobody understands me."

The older a teenager gets, the more many parents tend to relate at a maintenance level. We talk about the tasks that keep life—and the household—running. "Don't forget this. Have you done that? How about . . . ? Don't. . . ."

Listening becomes harder. And with little casual, friendly conversation and even less intimate sharing, understanding becomes almost impossible.

As I worked with the material in this chapter, I began to feel a greater sense of compassion for teens. The young people on the following pages gave me a great gift. They helped me understand teenagers more fully, and renewed my sense of appreciation for the wonder and the wanderings of the teenage years. I hope you catch some of that same feeling.

Trying to Communicate

Teenagers struggle, says psychiatrist Robert Coles,

> not only with the body's urges but with various
> social and economic strains on family life—

106

strains that have a direct bearing on adolescent sexuality. Parents who are themselves over- whelmed by joblessness or a precarious sur- vival; parents who are just barely getting by, often through second jobs, never mind the effort of both a mother and a father to stay employed; parents who are well-to-do but obsessed with their own lives, with their appearance, their social commitments, their travel plans and busi- ness obligations—such men and women are often not able to muster the interest and concern their not-so-young but still not fully grown children usually need, seek, urgently crave.[1]

Teenagers struggle to communicate what's going on inside of them. A sixteen-year-old girl tried to write out her frustration in a letter:

> . . . there's so much going on inside you, but you can't talk to anyone about it, even to your closest friend. I have this one girlfriend, and we used to be able to say anything to each other. But now even she—well, I can't talk to her about a lot of things.[2]

It is easy to get frustrated when someone can't seem to communicate clearly. For example, no matter how well- intentioned we are, we add to a stutterer's pain when we

---

1. Robert Coles and Geoffrey Stokes, *Sex and the American Teenager* (New York: Harper & Row Publishers, 1985).
2. Ibid.

rush to help him get out a difficult word. And we are often impatient with a teenager's attempts to tell us what's going on in his or her rapidly changing world.

"The world has changed so much in the last quarter century," observes sociologist Anthony Campolo, "that, when our kids accuse us of being out of touch with what's going on in the world, we must humbly confess that they're probably right. The time-honored directives that guided us through adolescence won't work for them."[3]

What Does It Feel Like to be a Teenager?

In a word of comfort and counsel to the parents of junior (and senior) highers, Harvard sociologist David Reisman argues:

> Social expectations for junior highers have changed so much and are in such flux that none of us know enough about them to properly guide our children through the precarious, formative early-teenage years. The folkways and mores that guided us older types through the junior-high rites of passage obviously do not apply to today's culture.[4]

Where, then, do we get the help we need? Who will tell us what it's like to be a teenager today?

Psychiatrist Robert Coles knows teens. "Adolescents," he says, "commonly feel themselves in the presence of an

---

3. *Youthworker,* Spring 1987.
4. Ibid.

enormous internal energy suddenly exerting itself. . . . Out of nowhere, it seems, the body is visited by this transforming presence."[5]

Teenagers long for understanding, and have an enormous capacity to reach out to others with that same understanding, as you can see in this letter from a young man to Dr. Coles:

> My dad can get down on this generation—mine! He'll sound off; he'll say we're selfish, and we've lost the values, the important values, of the older generation. But then minutes later he'll be telling me that he's not so proud of some of the things he did when he was my age; and he thinks we show more respect for each other, even if sometimes we don't always respect older people. (He means that we argue, he and I do!) Once he told me that he wasn't brought up to think about women the way guys like me do, and it was vice versa back then. "We were scared of each other; we didn't really have *friends* of the opposite sex," is the way he said it to me.
>
> Now that's changed! I can talk with girls I'm not dating—I mean, be real friendly with them. . . .

Today's teens are not about to be bought. They have a penetrating ability to see the difference between genuine, patient caring and look-alike substitutes.

---

5. Coles and Stokes, *Sex and the American Teenager.*

A Search for Intimacy

In these letters from teens, the search for intimacy comes through very clearly.

Society draws young people at lightning speed into the wider world—the away-from-home world. The all-important world of a small cluster of friends. They search for an intimacy that is harder and harder to find at home—or may never have been there in the first place.

With their search for intimacy comes an awakened sexuality. "The reality," says psychologist Dr. Richard Parsons, "is that adolescents are, will be, and *should be* sexually awakened."[6]

"With or without parental sanction, teen sexuality is a fact of life,"[7] observe psychotherapist Patricia Doyle and David Behrens.

Girls long to be close to someone. Boys, though they would hesitate to admit it, want to be held.

Like so many in the adult world, they feel that loving someone means having sex with them. And the difficult task of letting someone into the more intimate parts of their lives gets reduced to letting someone share the intimate parts of their bodies.

The Illusion of Intimacy

Youth counselors Mike Yaconelli and Jim Burns note:

---

6. Richard D. Parsons, *Adolescents in Turmoil, Parents Under Stress* (Mahwah, New Jersey: Paulist Press, 1987).
7. Patricia Doyle and David Behrens, *The Child in Crisis* (New York: McGraw-Hill Book Company, 1986).

High school students are becoming more and more addicted to experience. They constantly need to have some activity to look forward to. Looking forward to the weekend, for instance, becomes the reason for putting up with school and parents during the week. But the weekend has to contain *activities*.

The most serious side effect of "experience orientation" is that high-school students are easy prey to the *illusion of intimacy*. In other words, they easily mistake a relationship of *experience* for a relationship of *quality*.

This most often occurs in a relationship with someone of the opposite sex. Because high-school students are so susceptible to the sexual, it is easy for them to become involved with someone from the opposite sex and (as a result of the lack of sexual mores) suddenly experience intimacy so powerful and overwhelming that everything else in life seems dull and insignificant.

The experience of intimacy is addictive to the adolescent. It isn't unusual for high-school students to lose interest in everything except their relationships with boyfriends or girlfriends.[8]

What do teenagers' search for intimacy and their all-too-often willingness to settle for the *illusion* of intimacy say to parents?

---

8. Jim Burns and Mike Yaconelli, *High School Ministry* (Grand Rapids, Michigan: Zondervan Publishing House, 1986).

It suggests we must help our teenagers see that genuine intimacy happens slowly, in small, often difficult, risky steps. But we also must help them see that real intimacy is so special it is worth all the effort.

To do this we need to practice intimacy by being more open with our teens about our own struggles. They don't need all the intimate details, but they need to know that we are sometimes fearful and uncertain—that we are *real*.

And we need to cherish every opportunity for intimacy. Listen carefully to every question. Answer *slowly*. Quick, easy answers are seldom helpful—and they often demean the seriousness of both the question and the questioner.

What Teens Really Want

"Each stage of the psycho-social development of a youngster," explains sociologist Anthony Campolo, drawing on the observations of fellow sociologist Erik Erikson, "carries with it certain privileges and responsibilities." He points out that when young people assume privileges and responsibilities which belong to a stage of development that is beyond them, they often become emotionally disturbed and psychologically disoriented. Put simply, junior high kids often fall apart when they have the freedom to do all the things their parents seem all too willing to allow them to do. Very few of today's authority figures keep them from what they want to do, but these adolescents cannot exercise their freedom without inordinate fear and trepidation. Consequently, studies show that high school graduates looking back on their junior high years wish their parents had asked more questions of them and exercised more restraints on their behavior.[9]

It is all too much a part of modern parenting to stand back and give teens "the freedom to do what they want to do, to be pretty much what they want to be."

Robert Coles says:

> I wonder whether this inclination to stand apart, so to speak, on the part of many parents who have adolescent children is not a serious mistake—a misreading of what adolescents want and require, and maybe in some instances a rationalization to relieve some of us of a responsibility, thereby sparing us time for ourselves. Years of work with adolescents persuade me that they are the last ones in the world to want a freedom, a sense of privacy and autonomy that deprives them of the advice and counsel, the warm support and understanding of their parents, and, for that matter, of others (teachers, doctors) who are older and might have a good deal to say about some of the difficulties that confront a person of 15 or 16 or 17.[10]

---

9. *Youthworker,* Spring 1987.
10. Coles and Stokes, *Sex and the American Teenager.*

6

How to Talk to Your Teenagers— and Be Heard

For thirty-three years the doctor was chief of surgery at Children's Hospital of Philadelphia. For thirty-three years he talked with parents about their children's upcoming surgery. Patiently, carefully, he explained the planned procedures—and the risks.

Every anxious parent knew the doctor was being very honest. He understood their agony—and their doubts. And he didn't cheapen them by offering easy platitudes. They sensed his compassion, too. Above all, they trusted him, and somehow that made each family crisis more bearable.

Trying to Turn the Tide

Today that doctor speaks from a different platform. He is the nation's doctor, Surgeon General C. Everett Koop. For months now his subject has been AIDS. When he speaks, the almost brutal honesty is still there, as well as the integrity and the compassion.

He still speaks to parents, pleading, this time, for

their participation in turning the tide of this deadly disease:

> From my viewpoint, as a public health officer, I tell people that when they have sex with someone, they're also having sex with *everyone else* with whom *that* person has ever had sex. Naturally, if the "everyone else" is only you ... you're very well protected from disease ... and from a lot of other unpleasant surprises as well.
>
> This all seems to be information that is clear enough and straightforward enough to tell children.... Yet, many adults ... are having trouble coming to terms with it all.
>
> The more I've thought about this phenomenon, the more I've come to believe that the difficulty is not in the facts themselves concerning sexuality, human reproduction, and AIDS. The difficulty is in the *significance* of those facts relative to the totality of a *sensitive and affirmative* human relationship.
>
> Such a relationship will include some fulfilling sexual activity, but it is not defined *only by* that activity. There's much more to a loving, caring, respectful, and tolerant human relationship than just "good sex." A relationship devoid of love and responsibility is like a piece of pie that's all crust and no filling, and young people ought to be advised of that.
>
> Novelists call it "true love." Sociologists call it "marital fidelity." The Surgeon General calls it "monogamy." But whatever you call it, we all

want that well-rounded, balanced, loving, and fully considerate relationship . . . a relationship that's enriched by sex, not overwhelmed by it or devoid of it either.

Such a relationship is an ideal . . . but "real life" isn't always like that. It's imperfect . . . it's give-and-take.

Grown-ups know and come to accept human imperfection. But children don't . . . and won't.

Without a compassionate understanding of the imperfect nature of many human relationships, a child's education will be . . . itself . . . very imperfect.

So if parents are to educate their children about human relationships—sexual and otherwise—they must first understand and accept the nature of their *own*. For many, that's hard to do.

Parents—and adults in general—are not very good about talking *to each other* about their sexuality. They feel frustrated, guilty, and even angry because they are unable to do the thing that they know—intellectually and emotionally—they *should* do.

But they can't.

Is it any wonder, then, that many parents have difficulty telling children about the full-dimensional nature of an ideal human relationship?

Nevertheless, I want parents to try. I want parents to do this with compassion . . . with respect and with love . . . and with some understanding, not just of the child who's *listening* ... but also of the adult who is *speaking.*

It remains my sincerest wish that the *parents* of this country will be the primary teachers of sex and human relations to the *children* of this country.

I say that, knowing full well that many parents simply can't do it. But the task should not therefore be left, by default, to the movies ... to television ... or to the street corner. We can't do that, and still protect the millions of young lives that are at risk of AIDS.

My only hope is that every American who ... reads my message, will believe it and do his or her part to stop the spread of AIDS ... to protect and save the lives of people at risk, including and especially our unsuspecting young people ... and that they will help return sexuality to its rightful place in the spectrum of human experience: have it again be a *part* of the total complex of human, caring, interpersonal relations.[1]

On Talking to Your Kids About Sex, AIDS ... or Anything Else

Talking to your kids about AIDS must be part of talking to them about their sexuality.

We've always known that we *should* talk to them about sexual activity. Now the Surgeon General is telling us that

---

1. From a speech delivered by Surgeon General C. Everett Koop to the Joint Session on AIDS of the California Legislature, March 5, 1987.

117

we *must*. It's as if AIDS is forcing parents and kids to talk. Because there isn't a vaccine to prevent AIDS, or a drug to cure it, AIDS has put every teenager at risk.

That puts a lot of pressure on us parents. So we take the pressure seriously. We work hard at getting our facts straight. We go over and over what we plan to say. Now we're fearful, but we're ready.

But the truth is that parent-to-teen talk can't begin with AIDS—or even with sexuality.

Most "sex talks" make kids feel as if Mom or Dad is prying. And our best efforts are likely to be met with:

- Boredom. "Mom, I *know* all that stuff. We learn it in school."

- Verbal conformity. "Sure, Dad. What kind of guy do you think I am? I don't do that stuff."

  A lot of kids give parents this line. They tell themselves that "nobody tells their parents what's *really* going on. Besides, they don't have any way of knowing what I'm doing when I'm not at home."

- Resistance. "I haven't got time to talk about this stuff."

- Outright rejection. This is expressed in a variety of ways, from loud, angry words to a blunt refusal to listen.

As parents, it is easy for us to *expect* our kids to listen to us because of *who we are*. After all, we're parents: older, wiser, in control (we think). Or we expect to be heard by our kids because of *what we've done for them*. We've sacrificed in order to provide for them. Mere gratitude—or even common courtesy—requires that they listen, or so we often think.

It seems as if the older kids get, the less they listen. And that's a constant source of frustration—even anger—for concerned parents.

Our frustration is a direct result of the fact that we have been successful parents. We've taken a parent's primary task to heart: raising a child who is increasingly independent. And we've done it well. But with that success, we must increasingly surrender the right to *demand* attention or certain kinds of behavior.

Now we have to *win* the right to be heard.

And we win that right by building significant relationships with our children. If you want to be, or to *continue to be*, a primary influence in your child's life, you must have a solid, open relationship with that child.

"But I don't know how to build that kind of relationship," is no excuse. The stakes are too high. We all have to start. Don't let yourself feel inadequate. Don't be intimidated. From personal experience, let me assure you that there are no experts around to tell you how to relate to *your* kids. But I can offer you some insights that can help. In the end, it will be trial and some error—and every now and then a resounding success.

Enter Their World

Get to know kids and their world. That will take time and effort. You'll hear things you don't really want to hear, and maybe do things you don't really want to do. You'll take time for things that only make sense because you're seriously trying to understand another generation.

Rereading chapter 5 is a start. That chapter's letters from teens are full of the feelings of what it is like to be young. Let yourself experience those feelings. Let them touch you deeply.

So much of a teenager's world is made up of music. Constant music. Loud music. Sometimes disturbing music. When there's a teenager in the home, perhaps more parent-teen battles are fought over music than any other subject.

And because it is *his* music, or *her* music, it is perhaps the best bridge into their world, the best way to demonstrate that you care about the things your kids care about.

Listen to their music, not to criticize or compare, but just to listen. Just to show you're interested.

When teens mention some new artist, instead of saying "Who?" try responding with, "Tell me about him/her/them." Your "Who?" is a turn-off to kids. In your teenager's mind, when you don't know the rock stars who populate their world, that's one more confirmation to them that you really aren't interested in them.

Mike Warnke, a friend and sensitive youth counselor, told me:

> Kids really love it when their parents find value in what they do. But it's tough to start this process when your kids are fifteen or sixteen, because they've already become used to rejecting you. The first time you say, "I want to listen to one of your records," they're likely to say, "Get out of here." Your best effort at trying to let them know you want to understand their world will seem like an intrusion.

Parents tell me all the time that they have tried what I've been saying and it didn't work. I ask them how many times they tried. "Twice," they often say.

It takes more than that. Much more. Because you've already lost their confidence, it's going to take a while to get it back. But with patience, I believe it can be done.

You'll stumble in this process of getting acquainted with your own kids. Sure, you'll make some dumb mistakes. No doubt about it. Your kids might even roar with laughter. But all the time, they'll be getting the message that you are interested.

Talking About Feelings

The other way, maybe the best way, into a teenager's world is to talk about feelings. Teens know what feelings are. They have them all the time. Good feelings. Bad feelings. Happy feelings. Sad feelings. Confused feelings. Blah feelings.

Feelings come mostly in torrents. Someone said that "being a teenager is like having a caffeine high all the time."

Parents seem to want to ask *why* questions. "Why do you want to do this or that?" And kids find *why* questions hard to answer, because they may not know why. In many cases it never occurred to them to ask why they were doing a particular thing.

Don't get trapped into debating with your teenager, or arguing over matters of content. If you talk only about

121

content—and things, and issues, and facts—you'll some-times get verbal conformity and agreement. But that's easy for kids to give, if only to get you off their backs. It may do absolutely nothing to bring about change in your relationship or their life-style.

Deal with feelings. At any point in your relationship— or nonrelationship—with your teenager, you can get right to the heart of things by asking, "How do you feel about. . . ?" Be careful you don't presume how they feel or give even a hint that there is a right or a wrong feeling. Feelings simply are. And they need to be expressed.

You'll find some helpful "feelings" questions on pages 129, 130.

What Is Important in a Teen's World?

"Everybody's doing . . ." or "everybody's wearing. . . ." Every generation of teens can fill in the blanks with the "in" things of their era.

"Things" are always changing. But the big pressures kids face seem to remain much the same:

"Will I be accepted?"

Added to this age-old concern, today's teens face a new pressure; if they are not sexually active, they are out of step with "everybody else."

"What do I look like?"

Growing teens feel as if "everybody's looking at me" so much of the time. "They're all star-ing!"

This concern is expressed in two ways:

1. "My body." Everybody—teens *and* adults—
    has felt afraid to be seen in a bathing suit.
    And teens, more than anyone else, have parts
    of their bodies they don't like.

2. "My clothes." This is another source of
    parent-teen arguments. "How could you
    wear that?" a parent asks as the teenager is
    about to go out the door. What a teenager
    hears is, "You can't do *anything* right." A
    parent says, "That looks awful." The teen-
    ager hears, "*You* look awful."

"How coordinated am I?"

"Do I fit with the athletic crowd—girls or
boys—or do I belong with the nerds in the
library?"

Today's teen faces conflicting pressures. "How do I fit
into the crowd?" is an ever-present concern, always
doing battle with that other major concern, "How do I be
me?"

The parent-teen battleground needs to become a place
of listening, caring, and affirmation. There will *always* be
some battles. That is part of growing up. And parents
must be parents—*not* "best friends."

All of us need to look for opportunities for affirmation.
A very wise junior high school principal once advised the
parents of incoming seventh graders, "There are difficult
years ahead for your teenager. And you have *one single*

task. Find one thing your son or daughter does well. I don't care what it is, but find it. Then affirm them in that thing . . . even if you can't find anything else to affirm."

I'd like to add, *"Especially* if you can't find anything else to affirm."

Find something your teenager likes to do . . . some activity in which he (or she) will let you share.

Something. Anything. As long as it's something they want to do, and you're willing to try it. You don't have to be good at it. This isn't a competition.

This is especially important counsel for dads. Most dads spend all day being *productive.* Not wasting time. When they get home they have a long list of projects waiting. A son's or daughter's wishes can easily be seen as interruptions—and unplanned-for activities become a "waste of time."

Relationships are built on the interruptions and the wasted times. It is an especially significant way of saying that you really do care.

Begin today to practice being available.

A friend told me about spending time with his small son. This busy dad offered to do what the little boy wanted to do. He envisioned reading a book together, or something else that was "productive."

Instead the boy said, "I want to go out in the backyard and dig for worms and pill bugs." And so they did. Productive work by adult standards? No. Productive work in building a dad-son relationship? A hundred times, yes.

Try saying, "I'd really like to spend some time with you."

"Why, Dad? What for?"

"Oh, nothing! I'd just like to be with you, doing something you'd like to do."

Then let your son or daughter call the shots. Pull back from making the decisions.

Don't Be Discouraged

Like your initial attempt at listening to your kids' records, this may not work at first. You might have to suggest doing something together several times before your son or daughter will believe that you really *don't* have some hidden agenda, something you want to talk about. Keep trying. You gain ground in the relationship with every sincere try.

Winning a hearing is not a one-time thing. It will take serious, sustained effort. But if you've got something to say, and if you really want to be heard, that effort is absolutely essential.

Having another adult support and encourage you in the process can be very helpful. With your spouse, or an adult friend, talk about ideas for building a relationship with your teenager. As you talk, try to plan specific steps you want to take in order to:

- Be *with* your teenager in some way.

- Be a better listener—instead of an interrupter.

- Listen for—and even seek out—feelings.

- Share your feelings.

- Not make quick judgments or jump to conclusions.

Now that you're talking . . .

It's Time to Talk About Sex

Taking the time to win a hearing—*takes time*. But in the end, it opens the door to talk about things your kids really need to hear.

To make your part of the "sex talk" just a little easier, here are twelve steps for talking about sex that I've gathered from doctors, parents, and youth counselors. When you're ready to talk to your kids—*or your kids are ready to talk to you*—it would be helpful to look at these twelve steps again.

Each day, for twelve days, read one of the steps and spend ten to fifteen minutes quietly thinking about that step, and committing yourself to living it out with your family.

(For sources of quotations in this section, *see* the endnotes on page 132.)

Step One

Recognize that parents are important to kids.

Kids want to hear about sex information, as well as sexual attitudes and values, from their parents.

"Kids who can talk about sex with their more approachable parent are usually significantly *less* likely to have had intercourse than those who find it hard."[A]

Step Two

Recognize that you can't dictate behavior you can't control.

This is why a dialogue with your teen is so important. Ultimatums won't work.

"We must give [them] the skills to deal with

environmental pressures when the moment comes, usually in the absence of guiding adults."[B]

"Teenagers are not fools and tend to volunteer information about their sex lives only when they already have some reason to believe that they won't be met with chilly disapproval."[C]

Step Three

Recognize that you don't have to be a sex expert, or be totally at ease.

It is okay to feel uncomfortable. It is even okay to be upset, or somewhat frightened and anxious. But it is not okay to allow these feelings to be the excuse preventing any attempts at discussion.

"It is more important that the information be honest and accurate and presented in the form of a dialogue rather than a lecture.

"The fact that [parents] are willing to discuss what they do know, and be willing to seek advice for what they don't, will prove helpful."[E]

Step Four

Recognize that kids need good role models.

Kids need to see evidence that their parents love and care for each other and are comfortable in showing affection.

"Parents also need to begin to feel comfortable with their own sexuality so that they can model responsible sexual behavior and attitudes for their adolescents."[E]

Step Five

Be prepared for the fact that emotions—yours and your teenagers'—are bound to be strong when you talk about sex.

When your teenager reacts emotionally to what you are saying, you are no longer dealing with an issue. Now you are dealing—or need to deal—with *feelings*.

"Sexual warnings given in an anxious or angry tone of voice using judgmental language imply suspiciousness, distrust, and a fear of sexuality which the adolescent may greet with outright anger, oppositional behavior, or total social withdrawal from appropriate interaction."[C]

Step Six

Develop sensitivity.

Most teens don't seem to see premarital sex in terms of morality or immorality. They see it as a route to acceptance, intimacy, and belonging—qualities they are trying desperately to experience and understand. Parents who are aware of this are less likely to enter into a conversation on sex in a judgmental tone.

"Even if the kids are dead wrong, we need to listen to them."[F]

Step Seven

Don't criticize.

When parents criticize actions, kids often don't hear the criticism as something to be corrected. With their often fragile sense of self-worth, they are too busy hearing, "How could you be that kind of person?"

"Parents can pass on the message 'We may not think what you're doing is a good idea—but you still can come to us. We are still here for you.' "[D]

Step Eight

Encourage teens to share feelings.

Try asking questions that call for "feeling" answers, rather than for facts. Here are some suggestions:

Before a first date with a new person:

"How do you feel about this date?"

"You really look great. How do you feel about tonight?"

Before a really BIG date:

"I was really scared when I went out on a big date like this. How do you feel?"

Anytime:

"How are you feeling about that argument at school the other day? You seemed pretty discouraged at the time."

About sex . . . and AIDS:

"How do you feel when kids at school start talking about sex . . . or AIDS?"

"How would you feel if a good friend got AIDS?"

[After seeing something on TV about AIDS] "How does all this AIDS stuff make you feel?"

Most of us ask factual questions. It takes practice to ask "feeling" questions. These questions are meant to help you see what we're talking about. The answers to "feeling" questions often come more slowly. Teach yourself to wait for them.

If you absolutely cannot voice your feelings or concerns, you *could* try writing a letter. Teenagers are very letter and note oriented. You could say something like this:

> I'm not very good at communicating. In fact, I'm really scared about how you'll receive this. But I hope this note can at least open the door to help us share feelings without getting angry at each other.

Then go on from there—always keeping in mind that your goal is to open up *face-to-face* conversation.

Step Nine

Be specific.

Parental communication about sex is generally so vague or so limited that it has no impact.

"One young person told me recently, 'My dad told me not to do it, but he never told me *why* not to do it and when I did it I was disappointed. I wish he had explained his opinion to me.' "[F]

Step Ten

Share your own experiences and feelings.

As honestly as you can, be prepared to share some of your own teenage fears and failures. It can help to bridge the gap and make you a real person.

"[A] typical adolescent experience is the perception of being alone or misunderstood—that is, feeling

130

that no one else has had similar or the same experiences."[B]

Step Eleven

Set limits.

"At times [parents] set no limit at all—there is not a 'don't' expressed. The adolescent, however, picks up on this message and superficially may enjoy it, but also becomes enraged at his or her parents for lack of protection and empathy, empathy which encourages a helpful dialogue."[C]

"The awareness of parental guidelines is crucial to teenagers—because sexuality is a new and uncharted sea where there are no past boundaries and no memories to draw on."[D]

Step Twelve

It's never too late to start.

It's never too late to start communicating more openly, sensitively, and more clearly.

The most important step you can take is saying the first words. Don't wait for questions about sex. You must begin the discussion.

Remember that the gift of a patient, listening ear is the greatest gift you can give your son or daughter.

On Talking About AIDS

If you have children who are preteens (and not sexually active), there's no need for a formal "AIDS talk." I suggest that you respond to their questions about AIDS; repeat the question to be sure you understand. Then answer as factually as you can, using the material in chapters 2 through 4, and the information on grade school AIDS teaching programs in chapter 8.

If the subject comes up in conversation or on TV, you could ask, "What have you heard at school about AIDS?" or, "What are the kids saying about AIDS?"

If your kids are teens, or if they are sexually active, you can give them any of the information in this book—and you need to.

Endnotes to Chapter 6
A. Robert Coles and Geoffrey Stokes, *Sex and the American Teenager* (New York: Harper & Row Publishers, 1985).
B. Marion Howard, Ph.D., "How the Family Physician Can Help Young Teenagers Postpone Sexual Involvement," *Medical Aspects of Human Sexuality*, Vol. 19, No. 6, June 1985.
C. Jean Van De Polder, M.D., "Why Parents' Sexual Warnings to Adolescents Backfire," *Medical Aspects of Human Sexuality*, April 1980.
D. Patricia Doyle and David Behrens, *The Child in Crisis* (New York: McGraw-Hill Book Company, 1986).
E. Richard Parsons, Ph.D., *Adolescents in Turmoil, Parents Under Stress* (Mahwah, New Jersey: Paulist Press, 1987).
F. Jim Burns and Carol Bostrom, *Handling Your Hormones* (Laguna Hills, California: Merit Books, 1984).

7

Is There Such a Thing as "Safe Sex"?

Television commercials now proclaim loudly, "The Surgeon General says, 'The best protection—barring abstinence—is the use of a condom.' "

That quote is accurate, unquestionably. But it's not the whole story. It is only a part of what Surgeon General Koop has said.

Here is more of his statement:

> AIDS is no longer the concern of any one segment of society: it is the concern of us all. No American life is in danger if he/she or their sexual partners do not engage in high-risk sexual behavior or use shared needles or syringes to inject illicit drugs into the body.
>
> The most certain way to avoid getting the AIDS virus and to control the AIDS epidemic in the United States is for individuals to avoid promiscuous sexual practices, to maintain mu-

tually faithful, monogamous[1] sexual relationships and to avoid injecting illicit drugs.

Doctor Koop's Message

If you're young and you haven't yet achieved a
mutually faithful, monogamous relationship—
what this audience calls marriage—then you
should by all means take the best possible precautions against disease by abstaining. Period.
That's my advice to youngsters, and I don't think
there's any better advice you can give.

If you are an adult and have a faithful and
loving partner—and you are one yourself—then
sexuality is a part of that loving relationship
and there is no need for abstinence.[2]

At the National Press Club, Koop said:

In order to end the chain of transmission of this
disease once and for all, we need to teach our
young people the facts about AIDS and about
their own sexuality. The objective is to make
them a lot more responsible in their relationships than their elders have been. . . .[3]

---

1. *Monogamous* means being married to one person at a time.
2. From a speech Dr. Koop delivered to the National Association of
   Religious Broadcasters, Washington, D.C., February 2, 1987.
3. From the Surgeon General's speech to the National Press Club,
   Washington, D.C., March 24, 1987.

On another occasion he said, "I believe children should be taught to be abstinent until they grow up, assume the role of a responsible adult, and find a mutually monogamous relationship. That doesn't seem to be too farfetched. In fact, it was once the norm for this country, and a return to such a norm would ensure the end of sexually transmitted AIDS."[4]

He repeated the same message in a speech at Children's Hospital of Philadelphia, then added pointedly:

> My second message is for people who don't yet have a faithful, monogamous relationship for whatever reason; unless you know with absolute certainty that neither you nor your partner is carrying the AIDS virus, you must use caution.
>
> Remember . . . when you have sex with someone, you're also having sex with everyone else with whom that person has had sex.
>
> And when you consider the long incubation period for the AIDS virus, we're talking about that person's history of sexual relations going back five years[5] or perhaps longer.[6]

---

4. From a speech presented by the Surgeon General to the Annual Meeting of the National School Boards Association, San Francisco, California, April 4, 1987.
5. Dr. Koop and others have stated that it could be ten years or more between infection and the point at which the person carrying the virus contracts an AIDS-related disease.
6. Presented by the Surgeon General as the Pasquariello Lecture at the Children's Hospital of Philadelphia, April 8, 1987.

Expanding the Campaign

As the virus has spread to new segments of the population, the Surgeon General and the Public Health Service have enlarged the focus of their educational campaign.

"When we first began to confront the AIDS epidemic," says Dr. Koop, "the people at highest risk were homosexual and bisexual men and IV drug abusers, male and female.

"But nowadays we're receiving more and more reports of the AIDS virus occurring among heterosexual men and women who are not IV drug abusers. In fact, their heterosexual activity seems to be their only risk factor."[7]

Make no mistake. The Surgeon General's counsel is crystal clear, and it is addressed to every sexually active person, male or female, heterosexual or homosexual, younger or older.

The AIDS era demands changes in our nation's sexual practices. And our deep fears confirm those demands.

Diane Feinstein, the mayor of San Francisco, has declared, "We can no longer be a promiscuous society."[8]

Changing any habit pattern is difficult, and that is particularly true for the young, who are just beginning to explore the so-called sexual revolution and taste its heady fruit.

---

7. Lecture at Children's Hospital.
8. Mayor Feinstein made her statement on "National Town Meeting on AIDS" on the ABC television network.

Encouraging Change

How do you bring about changes in sexual behavior? "It's a three-step process," says Dr. Neil Schram.[9] "People must understand that there is a risk, then believe that they can do something to lower that risk, and finally, choose to practice the low-risk behavior."

Throughout these pages I have sought to make that message very clear.

The second message—one I hope is equally clear—is that something can be done to lower, or even eliminate, the risk.

The real test of how well you and I have done our job will be that the young come to see *for themselves* that AIDS is a risk to them if they are sexually active. And they must also come to see that they can do something to lower, or eliminate, that risk.

For those not yet sexually active, lowering or eliminating the risk of AIDS seems easier. Not *easy*, mind you, but at least a little easier.

For those who are already active, the task of helping them *want* to lower or eliminate the risks is a most demanding one.

In the light of this difficult task, it is no surprise that many parents settle for some "assurance" of risk reduction from their kids and heave a sigh of relief.

But before you consider that option, I want you first to walk with me down the much more difficult path of risk *elimination*. This road is not an easy one, but I assure you that it is well worth the effort.

---

9. Dr. Schram is an internist and the former chairman of the Los Angeles City/County AIDS Task Force.

The Search for Closeness

The experts say it. Teens themselves say it: They are looking for closeness. For touch. For affection.

That search runs like a scarlet cord through the letters and comments of the teens in chapter 5. The only way some teens know how to be close to someone else is through sex.

Teenagers need models of closeness that don't involve sex. If your relationship with your teen is an open one, you can help him/her remember moments of closeness in the family, or times when they felt close to a friend. Talk about what made that closeness. Was it something physical? Sometimes the answer would be yes, but more often than not, closeness happens when one person cares enough about another to share some little piece of himself or herself that wouldn't otherwise be known.

Sometimes you feel close as you laugh together. Other times silence seems to bring a feeling of closeness. There are times, too, when we feel close to people who listen to us so intently they seem to shut out everything and everyone else. Closeness can happen when you say things like, "I thought about you and that test today. Did everything go okay?" or, "How do you feel about it?"

Real closeness doesn't happen every day. But when it does it is very special. Slow down, and find more of those moments with your teenager. Then, remembering those moments and talking about them later can help your young person see that sex is meant to be a wonderful expression of closeness—but it is not the only way to find closeness; nor, for the young, is it the best way.

Pleasing One's Partner

Many a young girl feels as if sexual intercourse is essential in order to "please" her friend.

You can affirm that it is wonderful to want to please another person. But learning to *really* please a friend takes time and effort. A person can spend a lifetime learning the simple things that give a friend joy.

Help your teenager develop a sensitivity to small pleasures. Talk about the things a friend "really likes," especially those you don't have to buy.

The goal is to help young people learn how to deepen relationships without sacrificing themselves in the process.

A Good Self-Image

There is perhaps nothing so crucial, or so difficult, for many young people as the development of a good self-image. In a teenage world of constant comparisons, of "in" groups and outsiders, where humor can be biting and survival often goes to the fittest, or the boldest, it is tough to feel good about oneself. And when home adds to those pressures, the burden is almost unbearable.

Our adult world isn't all that different. When we come home at the end of the day we often need someone to affirm us, to tell us—or better still, show us—that we are special.

We need a little space at the end of the day, maybe some time just to be quiet. But we also need to find the energy to affirm the worth of our teens. That is part of what home and family are all about.

If and when our teenagers want to talk, they need our attention. That's a simple way we can say, "You are special to me." They need to hear our approval when they have done something special. And they need to hear our apologies when we have misjudged them or done something wrong.

We know what pressures and compromises are like. We know the strength it takes to hold the line in our adult world. And we know that that task is easier for us when we are feeling good about ourselves.

Let's do our best to give our teens that very special gift—the gift of self-worth.

What Does It Mean to Be "In Love"?

That's a tough question. One person describes it as a whole bunch of warm feelings. At the other end of the "in love" spectrum, true love could be defined as a rich collection of shared experiences.

The definition of *love* becomes critical in the AIDS epidemic since, in the minds of the young, being in love opens the door to much more intimate sexual experiences.

Sociologists report that the average person is in love from three to five times before marriage. In the search for Miss or Mr. Right, the young seem to be able to recover fairly quickly from one broken relationship and continue the search.

Can our young people really know when Miss or Mr. Right comes along?

Here are some points to talk about: *Good, warm feelings* must be at least a part of love. I'd hate to think that falling in love was nothing more than establishing a straightforward partnership agreement. But love must be more than warm feelings.

Being in love combines the *closeness,* the *pleasing and being pleased,* and the *increasing sense of self-worth* we've been talking about. At the very least, these things make good soil in which true love can grow. Without them, there is little chance of lasting love.

True love ought to involve *increasing trust and openness between partners.* That is one of the important reasons love leads logically to marriage. In marriage, we are making a public commitment to stay together in an intimate relationship. The permanence of marriage was meant to provide a kind of security—a place where we can risk being known as we really are, without risking the relationship itself. It is a place where either partner can fail, without the relationship failing.

Tim Stafford, author of a widely read column for teens, feels that there is only one reliable test of "true love":

> Are you both ready and willing to have a wedding ceremony—to declare your commitment in front of family, friends and God? To live together, legally tied together, sharing everything?
>
> If you're not ready for that heady step, you can't be very sure that your love will last. Weddings aren't guaranteed, but they do pro-

vide the best test ever designed for separating big talkers from the truly committed.[10]

There is one more test worth looking at. It has stood for two thousand years as a description of true love:

> Love is always patient and kind; love is never jealous; love is not boastful or conceited; it is never rude and never seeks its own advantage; it does not take offence, or store up grievances. Love does not rejoice at wrongdoing but finds its joy in the truth; it is always ready to make allowances, to trust, to hope, and to endure whatever comes.[11]

It is easy to dismiss those words as "too idealistic," "impossible," "nobody can live like that." But there is great joy in the trying. The fact that even the most sensitive among us falls short of that kind of love is no reason to abandon the effort. It is only a reminder that true love doesn't just happen; it takes a lifetime of commitment to begin to experience its limitless depths and heights.

Helping teens understand being "in love" may call for sharing some of your own attempts to learn what love means. Lofty concepts become more real when we see someone else's efforts to live them out.

---

10. Tim Stafford, *How to Say No* (San Bernardino, California: Worldwide Challenge, 1986).
11. First Corinthians 13:4–7. Excerpt from THE NEW JERUSALEM BIBLE, copyright © 1985 by Darton, Longman & Todd, Ltd. and Doubleday & Company, Inc. Reprinted by permission of the publisher.

You've Got to Talk

If a young couple has been dating more than a few weeks, they had better talk seriously about what they will or won't allow sexually. They need to talk about a stopping point, and make sure that the ground rules are understood.

They also need to make sure that those ground rules are based upon a clear understanding of the risks involved in the various kinds of sexual activities.

Young people seem to feel that talking takes the spontaneity out of loving. But the reality of AIDS has made this kind of talk absolutely essential.

If they can't talk about ground rules, the safest thing is to get out of that relationship. The risk of continuing is too great.

Learning to Say No

The AIDS epidemic can be stopped. A lot of people think the best way to do that is to quarantine those people who are infected with the virus. But that simply relieves the rest of us of doing anything about the problem. And it assumes that it would be possible to quarantine every infected person.

The only real answer is self-quarantine. Ellen Goodman, a syndicated newspaper columnist, has said it clearly: "We can only stop the spread of AIDS at the border of our own lives."[12]

Saying no to anything can be difficult. Saying no to sexual intercourse is especially tough. You can help your

---

12. From Ms. Goodman's column in the *Los Angeles Times.*

teens know that they have the right to say no to sex without having to give any explanation for their decision.

Doctor Marion Howard offers these suggestions on how to say no:

> First say no, and keep repeating it. Surprisingly enough, that really does work. On the off chance that it doesn't work, however, tell the other person how continuing pressure makes you feel. You can say, "When you keep pressuring me after I've told you no, you make me angry" or, "It makes me feel you really don't care about me." Most often, this works if continued no's don't.
>
> If even that doesn't work, just get out of the situation entirely; remove yourself from the pressure to discuss it further, walk out of the room, if necessary.[13]

If saying no means your teenagers may not have transportation home, they need to know—in advance—that you will pay for a taxi ride home, or you will pick them up with no heavy questions asked on the way home.

Young people also need to know that other kids are saying no. Like all of us, they need support when they take a difficult stand. They see the risks of taking that stand. A close friend, and now and then, a parent, can give them the positive reinforcement they need.

---

13. Marion Howard, Ph.D., is Associate Professor, Department of Gynecology and Obstetrics, Emory University School of Medicine, and Clinical Director, Teen Services Program, Grady Memorial Hospital, Atlanta, Georgia. Reprinted from *Medical Aspects of Human Sexuality*, Vol. 19, No. 6, June 1986.

The Value of Compassion

Taking the time to read about AIDS and to seek out the latest information doesn't have to dominate family conversations, but the fact that you are aware and concerned can reinforce your family's sense of the risk of AIDS.

With your new knowledge, you and your family can also help perform a major task: You can help correct misinformation.

Setting the example of compassionate concern toward people with AIDS will help your teenager take this disease seriously, and see *people* with AIDS, rather than seeing a *disease* that infects people.

Your compassionate attitude will also affirm the fact that you are approachable when tough problems arise. It says that when the chips are down, you are committed to caring rather than criticizing.

Beyond the home, you and other members of your family might want to consider volunteering some time to help people with AIDS. There are buddy programs through which you could provide help and care for one person.[14] Hospices and home health care services for people with AIDS always need volunteers.[15] Check with a local doctor or public health office for programs like these in your community.

---

14. The City of Austin, Texas, is providing this kind of program through AIDS Services of Austin, P.O. Box 4874, Austin, TX 78765, phone 512-458-AIDS.

15. The Hospice of San Francisco offers a comprehensive manual on establishing a hospice. Ask for information on the *AIDS Home Care and Hospice Manual* from the Hospice of San Francisco, 401 Duboce Avenue, San Francisco, CA 94117, phone 415-861-8705.

If They Are Going to Have Intercourse

Let's change the subject for just a minute. Let's talk about teenage drinking.

Many parents have said to teenagers, "We can't watch you all the time, and we wouldn't want to. We've talked about the problems involved with alcohol, and we really hope you'll decide not to drink. But here is the absolute bottom line for us: If you drink, *don't ever drive.* Call us. We'll come and get you. And please don't ride in a car with a driver who has been drinking."

That's clear communication. It says, "You know the risks. You know how we feel. But we can't control you. You'll be making your own decisions. Because we could be talking about your life, don't let our concerns keep you from asking for help. We'll be there for you."

The attitude about sex has to be the same. "You know the risks. We've talked about them. You know the talks we've had about love and sex. But here is the bottom line: If you're going to have sex, you will need to ask your partner intimate questions about any previous sexual activity, and be absolutely sure you can trust the answers.

"And you'll need to be sure your partner, and any of his or her partners, have never shared someone's IV drug needles.

"When you think about it, you'll probably want to wait so that you can know more about the person and the possibility of AIDS infection—or be able to trust his/her answers more completely. If this doesn't convince you to abstain . . . use a condom."

That's the message kids have to hear. Their lives may depend on it.

Condoms and "Safe Sex"

Condoms cannot guarantee safe sex. Outside of a long-term monogamous relationship, in which both partners are *known* to be free of HIV, observes Professor Marcus Conant, M.D., of the University of California, San Francisco, there is no safe sex anymore.[16]

In a recent laboratory study of latex and natural-membrane condoms, Dr. Conant reported that "none of the viral agents passed through the latex, while there was occasional leakage in natural condoms." According to the U.S. Food and Drug Administration, one out of every five batches of condoms tested in laboratories by the government in mid-1987 failed to meet minimum standards for leakage. This and more information on condoms can be found in Questions 69–75 in Chapter 4.

Marsha Goldsmith, in the *Journal of the American Medical Association,* quotes the following condom use checklist developed by Robert Hatcher, M.D., M.P.H., Professor of Gynecology and Obstetrics at Atlanta's Emory University School of Medicine.

1. Use a condom every single time you have intercourse. There is no "safe" time with regard to transmitting disease.

2. Put the condom on as soon as erection occurs. Unprotected contact with any orifice—vagina, mouth, or rectum—is unsafe.

3. Roll the condom's rim all the way to the base of the

---

16. Marsha F. Goldsmith, "Sex in the Age of AIDS," *Journal of the American Medical Association*, Vol. 257, No. 17, May 1, 1987.

penis before insertion into the partner. If the condom lacks a reservoir tip, leave a small empty space at the tip to catch semen.

4. For lubrication, do not use petroleum jelly, vegetable shortening, or oil, because they may deteriorate the latex. Neither is saliva recommended. Sufficient lubrication is needed so the condom will not tear; if more lubrication is required, use water or spermicidal jelly or spermicidal foam, preferably containing nonoxynol 9.

5. After intercourse, hold on to the rim of the condom as the penis is withdrawn, being careful not to spill any semen. Withdraw the penis from the partner soon after ejaculation, because if the erection is lost the condom may slip off, allowing semen to escape.

6. Do not use a condom more than once. Dispose of it safely, so that no one (a youngster, for example) has access to it.

7. Store condoms in a cool, dry place. Do not keep them in a wallet or other hot place for a long time because heat can deteriorate the latex.

Obviously, we hope our young people will wait for marriage to experience a loving sexual relationship. But if your son is going to have sex, he must wear a condom—and wear it properly—for his own safety and that of his partner.

If your daughter is going to have sex, she must be prepared to insist that the boy wear a condom from the start to the finish of intercourse. And she must be prepared to provide the condom. That is a heavy burden to place on a girl, but it is reality. Most sexually active boys resist using a condom, and the majority of the condoms sold today are sold to women.

Few of us like this alternative. We wish fervently that we didn't have to think about things like teenage sexual activity . . . and condoms. But we have no choice. We must face the facts. The lives of our young people are at stake, and *none of us* is willing to risk that sacrifice.

That brings us back to where we started this chapter: "The Surgeon General says, 'The best protection—barring abstinence—is the use of a condom.' "

We've talked about what it could take to encourage abstinence—the only sure, absolutely safe protection. If abstinence is not possible for some of our young, we must face the fact that the condom is presently the only other protection available. It's that simple.

8

AIDS Education in School and Other Places

The young mother with AIDS looked into the face of her doctor. She could see comfort . . . and compassion. He was busy, yet he always seemed to find the time to be gentle.

But his answers to her questions were never the ones she wanted so desperately to hear. Her most recent bout with Pneumocystis carinii pneumonia (she now called it PCP because it was easier to say) was over. But she was still so weak. And she knew there would be another bout.

That was what ate at her insides; there would be another . . . and another. . . . Just yesterday she had tried to break through the doctor's gentleness with all the energy she could muster.

"Don't give me your kindness," she tried to raise her voice. "I don't want help. I want HOPE."

Her cry was more of deep sadness than anger. More of a plea than a scream.

The doctor had dropped his head, then reached out to take her hand. He didn't say anything. He couldn't. They both knew the almost unbearable truth: that there was no hope. She would last maybe a few months, but no more.

*   *   *

The teacher looked out into the faces of her students. Bright faces, some of them. Some still a little weary. "It's only the second class of the morning, Mrs. Marchuk," one of the boys had said only last week.

This morning when she came into the room there was more laughter than usual. Nervous laughter. Now it had turned to a silence she could feel. A silence more of apprehension than of interest. A good teacher knew the difference. And Mrs. Marchuk was *good*.

As she began passing out the new student guide on AIDS, she walked around the room, looking each student in the face. She often did this when they were about to begin a new unit of study. It helped her focus on the students as individuals rather than just as parts of a class. And it helped give her a sense of hope.

That was what made this ninth-grade class special— hope. They were open enough to ask honest, hard questions. And young enough to learn new, safer sexual attitudes.

There was hope in Mrs. Marchuk's classroom. Like no other class in that junior high that morning, *this* one was facing a life-threatening situation ... and discovering that, for them, there was hope.

*   *   *

Two scenes. Two realities. Each so vastly different from the other.

One—hopeless.

One—full of hope.

To stand by the bedside of a person with AIDS is to feel

a pain deeper than any pain you've felt before. You can't help but come away with a resolve to care more deeply and support more sacrificially every worthwhile effort to alleviate the pain of the dying and to find a cure for this dreaded condition.

The students in Mrs. Marchuk's classroom—and all the other classrooms of America—are so vulnerable. So adult one moment, so childish the next. So caught up in trying to understand and to cope with their sexual urges.

To hear what goes on in that classroom is to understand how important—how essential—sex education is. How important that it be done well. How important that it present a model of *responsible* sexual behavior. How important that parents act responsibly as supportive partners in this vital process.

Our Only Weapon

The Surgeon General said to parents, "Education . . . education . . . education. Right now, that's our *only* weapon against this dreadful disease. With your help, it can also be the *strongest* weapon we have."[1]

Then he went on to say more about this important and controversial subject:

> We have only a few years of grace to help a young child understand his or her sexuality before the onset of puberty.
>
> Also, a parent should handle this education

1. From a speech to the National Religious Broadcasters, Washington, D.C., February 2, 1987.

of the child, but experience has shown that a parent can never be the exclusive educator. The *best* educator . . . the *educator of choice* . . . yes, of course. But the *exclusive* educator, I doubt that.

I wish we *could* say that parents who want to can be in total control of a child's sex education. But we know that children do learn about sex from many unstructured and unplanned experiences.

When he talked about structured sex education classes, Dr. Koop observed:

I'd rather call [them] "Health and Human Development" [classes. They] can probably be taught beginning in kindergarten and first grade. And here I'm speaking of a curriculum that answers the common, everyday questions raised by young children, questions such as, "Where do babies come from?"

This kind of education can and should be nonthreatening . . . it can teach good values . . . it can help develop the child's own sense of personal responsibility . . . and it can strengthen the concept of "the family."

This kind of sex education should unfold according to the developmental age of children and to their different levels of awareness and curiosity. I don't see any reason to cling to a rigid schedule based on chronological age.

If the curriculum is well planned and thoughtfully carried out, then it will be possible to bring to the attention of the children the facts about sexually transmitted diseases—and AIDS in particular—along about the junior high school years . . . the years of early adolescence.

In Spite of the Critics

Some uninformed, inaccurate, and less-than-honest critics of my position believe that what I've just said is tantamount to the most heinous of activities. They say it means, for example, and I'm quoting now . . .

". . . sponsoring homosexually oriented curricula . . ."

". . . teaching buggery in the third grade . . ."

". . . providing condoms to eight-year-olds. . . ."

Nothing could be further from the truth.

Dr. Koop describes the development of his educational proposal this way:

I talked with the representatives of twenty-six groups in all. Most of them knew quite a bit about the health threat posed by AIDS. But what they were deeply troubled about were the moral and ethical issues raised by this disease.

Yes, we all agreed that the only real weapon we had to fight with at this time—since we lacked a vaccine or an effective drug—was the weapon of education.

154

That's where we all agreed. Where we had some differences of opinion was the *substance* and the *direction* of that education.

Everybody had said, yes, we should teach about the dangers posed by the AIDS virus.

Most people said, well, *maybe* we should teach about the methods by which AIDS is transmitted.

And quite a few people said that, of course, we might *possibly* teach young people something about their sexuality to begin with.

I listened to everybody and took very good notes.

You may recall that my entire report[2] is not very long. And I only devoted *ninety-two* words to the topic of education. But those ninety-two words have captured most of the attention of the media, of parents, of educators, and of public officials at all levels of government.

The reason is clear enough: The issue goes to the heart of each person's own system of moral and ethical values . . . or lack thereof.

I introduced the subject in a straightforward way. I said in my report:

Education about AIDS should start in early elementary school and at home so that children can grow up knowing the behavior to avoid to protect themselves from exposure to the AIDS virus. The threat of

---

2. The *Surgeon General's Report on AIDS.*

AIDS can provide an opportunity for parents to instill in their children their own moral and ethical standards.

Some people were unduly alarmed by that phrase, "early elementary school." Would that include kindergarten? I'm afraid so.

I know of good, caring approaches to sex education that can be used—and in fact *are* used—in kindergarten and first grade.

However, I recognize that it's more difficult to do and, therefore, I would be willing today, some four months after publication, to make that single change in the report . . . that is, I would agree, albeit reluctantly, to take out the word *early* and just let the sentence read, "Education about AIDS should start in elementary school."

I concluded the report with exactly the same thought. I said:

Education concerning AIDS must start at the lowest grade possible as part of any health and hygiene program. . . . There is now no doubt that we need sex education in schools and that it must include information on heterosexual and homosexual relationships. The threat of AIDS should be sufficient to permit a sex education curriculum with a heavy emphasis on prevention of AIDS and other sexually transmitted diseases.

156

And I would not change *any* of the words in that paragraph.[3]

Making the Message Clear

To make his message even clearer, in January 1987, Dr. Koop joined with Secretary of Education William J. Bennett in issuing this statement on the principles they felt should shape AIDS education:

> AIDS is a serious threat to our citizenry. Education has a fundamental role to play in teaching our young people how to avoid that threat. With the appropriate involvement and approval of parents and the local community, schools should *help* teach young people about the danger of AIDS.

Then it went on to state these four principles:

> 1. *Our young people deserve the best scientific information about this disease, and the ways in which it is transmitted.* The Federal Government has a responsibility to provide such information to local education authorities.
> 2. *As in other areas, decisions as to the proper timing, particular course content, and the like are fundamentally ones for states and*

---

3. From a speech by the Surgeon General to the Joint Session on AIDS of the California Legislature, Sacramento, California, March 5, 1987.

local communities to make. But if schools do teach sex education, such courses should include a discussion of the threat posed by AIDS. And as with sex education courses in general, it is especially important in a sensitive area like this one that school officials consult widely with parents, local public health officials and community members to determine when and how to introduce such material into the classroom.

3. *Young people must be told the truth—that the best way to avoid AIDS is to refrain from sexual activity until as adults they are ready to establish a mutually faithful, monogamous relationship.* Since sex education courses should in any case teach children why they should refrain from engaging in sexual intercourse, AIDS education should confirm the message that should already be there in the sex education curriculum. AIDS education (as part of sex education in general) should uphold monogamy in marriage as a desirable and worthy thing.

4. *AIDS education guided by these principles can help protect our children from this terrible disease. But an AIDS education that accepts children's sexual activity as inevitable and focuses only on "safe sex" will be at best ineffectual, at worst itself a cause of serious harm.* Young people should be taught that the best precaution is abstinence until it is possible

to establish a mutually faithful, monogamous relationship.

With regard to AIDS, science and morality teach the same lesson. The *Surgeon General's Report on AIDS* makes it clear that the best way to avoid AIDS is a mutually faithful, monogamous sexual relationship. Until it is possible to establish and maintain such a relationship, abstinence is safest.[4] (Emphasis added.)

The White House Position

Two weeks after the joint Bennett/Koop statement, the White House Domestic Policy Council issued a list of principles the president had adopted regarding the federal government's position on education about AIDS.

The memo contained, among other things, this declaration:

Any health information developed by the Federal Government that will be used for education should *encourage responsible sexual behavior— based on fidelity, commitment, and maturity, placing sexuality within the context of marriage.*

Any health information provided by the Federal Government that might be used in schools

---

4. "Statement on AIDS Education" issued January 30, 1987, by the Office of the Secretary, United States Department of Education, and signed by Secretary of Education William J. Bennett and Surgeon General C. Everett Koop, M.D.

should teach that *children should not engage in sex, and should be used with the consent and involvement of parents.*[5] (Emphasis added.)

What's Happening Across the Country?

A survey of seventy-three of the country's largest school districts conducted by the United States Conference of Mayors found that (as of December 1986) forty school districts were already providing AIDS education.[6] An additional twenty-four districts were planning educational efforts.

Grade Levels

Most school districts reported providing AIDS education in the junior and senior high school years (grades 7–12). Tenth-grade students (high school sophomores) are the primary focus, followed by seventh-graders, then ninth-graders.

Schools generally provided students at higher grade levels with more detailed AIDS information.

The survey results indicated that, at the grade school level:

---

5. "Memorandum for the Domestic Policy Council on the Subject of AIDS Education," issued by the White House, February 11, 1987.
6. A more detailed report on the survey from which this information has been drawn is available from the United States Conference of Mayors, 1620 Eye Street, N.W., Washington, D.C. 20006, phone 202-293-7330. Ask for AIDS Information Exchange, Vol. 4, No. 1, January 1987.

Information about AIDS is taught on a very general level and does not cover the specifics of transmission of the disease, high-risk behavior, or precautions to take in avoiding AIDS. This approach is consistent with other facets of elementary level education dealing with sex and STDs [Sexually Transmitted Diseases], where the emphasis is on educating students about individual hygiene and awareness of one's body.

Subjects Taught

At the secondary school level the medical facts about AIDS and how it is transmitted are taught in virtually all AIDS programs surveyed.

School districts were asked if they provided discussion of condom use, selection of sexual partners, avoidance of high-risk sexual activities, and abstinence.

Seventy-eight percent dealt with abstinence.[7] The other three risk-reduction options were discussed in 70 percent of the school districts with current programs.

Parental Permission

Only 45 percent of the school districts required parental permission prior to teaching students about AIDS.

---

7. The Anchorage, Alaska, School District offers a Refusal Skills Program, "How to Say No." For information write Anchorage School District, Health Services Department, P.O. Box 196614, Anchorage, AK 99519-6614, phone 907-333-9561.

Developing AIDS Programs

School districts have generally worked with outside organizations in developing their course of study on AIDS. Eighty percent worked with local and state health departments. Fifty percent drew on the help of community organizations (gay/bisexual service organizations, the American Red Cross, Planned Parenthood, YMCA, YWCA).

Only 31 percent of the districts worked with local PTAs. Thirty districts (47 percent) listed organizational assistance from clergy, state education agencies, student councils, health professionals, universities, and the Centers for Disease Control.

The "Values" Battle

School districts and teachers appear to be caught in a bind. In a classroom there are some students who are not sexually active, and their decision to abstain must be supported. But there are other students in that same classroom—perhaps a majority, depending on the school grade—who are sexually active, and at great risk of contracting AIDS.

Like the Surgeon General, as much as a teacher may want to—indeed must—proclaim abstinence as a viable option, he or she must also face the reality that young lives are at risk and if that risk cannot be eliminated by changed behavior, then it must at the very least be reduced.

However, that dilemma cannot cause the scales to tip

too easily away from abstinence, and toward "safe sex."

We must see to it that school districts continue to hold these two seemingly opposed positions in tension.

To accomplish this, parents need to be involved with the schools. But our efforts must be those of a friend rather than an enemy. We must be seen as offering cooperation and understanding, not battle and belligerence. School personnel must be treated as people who are well intentioned.

Educators do try to be responsive. As an example of attempts to reduce classroom pressure for students to go along with the group, here, from a new AIDS curriculum teachers' guide, are some suggestions for conducting an attitude-related discussion:

1. Student participation should be *voluntary*, and the choice of *whether or not to participate should be unrelated to the student's class grade.*

2. To *ensure anonymity*, names should not be placed on the work sheets.

3. No student should be *required* to share his or her views with others.

4. Any views expressed should not be labeled as "right" or "wrong" by the teacher. Discussion should examine values that *enhance the control of AIDS.*

5. The activity should be suited to the particular group of students. (For example, are the students mature enough to handle this activity? Is there sufficient trust within the classroom for open discussion?)

And the same guidebook urges community involvement:

> Most communities have strong interest in school education about AIDS. They generally support instruction, *but are often concerned about the exact nature of the course content.* This curriculum was written to be accepted by a broad spectrum of communities. Deliberate efforts were made to discuss the material discreetly and tactfully, as well as to be scientifically objective.
>
> *It is suggested that the curriculum be discussed with representatives of the local community.* Typically for the STD instructional area, community involvement in the curriculum process leads to strong support for teaching the subject. *Students should be encouraged to share their AIDS book with parents. This can address some of the concerns, fears, and questions that parents may have.*[8] (Emphasis added.)

The pendulum may be swinging away from valueless sex education. *Abstinence* is the strong emphasis of several new teaching programs. The Minneapolis-based

---

8. From *AIDS: What Young Adults Should Know* (Instruction Guide), copyright © 1987 by American Alliance for Health, Physical Education, Recreation, and Dance, 1900 Association Drive, Reston, VA 22091, phone 703-476-3400.

Search Institute[9] has recently released *Yes You Can: Affirming Sexual Abstinence Among Young Teens.* The book is described as "a guide for designing and introducing effective education in human sexuality for young adolescents." *Yes You Can*, with its emphasis on teaching affirmative values, was produced under a grant from the United States Department of Health and Human Services. Search Institute has also released *Values and Choices*, a course in human sexuality for seventh- and eighth-graders *and their parents.*

Strengthening the Impact

"An annual seminar or a week's worth of health class study on AIDS," observes Dr. Neil Schram, "is not sufficient to make a lasting impression on young people, especially those who have little or no exposure to sexual activity or drug use at the time of the lecture. What's needed is frequent counseling, perhaps monthly, preferably on a one-to-one basis, to encourage frankness and confidentiality."

The Seattle (Washington)–Kings County Chapter of the American Red Cross provides a training conference on AIDS communication for people who work with high school newspapers. This unique peer teaching program has proven very effective. Student journalists who participated are now informal counselors to other students.

Program coordinators report that students often receive

---

9. Search Institute, 122 West Franklin Avenue, Suite 525, Minneapolis, MN 55404-9990, phone 612-870-9511.

phone calls from young people asking, "What did you mean when you said . . . ?" or, "I'm scared. Where do I get help?"[10]

Church youth groups, YMCAs, YWCAs, and other community service groups could offer classes for parents and youth.

A Legislative Response

California State Senator Gary Hart authored legislation requiring the State Department of Education to purchase and distribute informational materials on AIDS prevention to all school districts that offer AIDS instruction in grades 7 through 12.

The actual bill calls for those materials to include "at a minimum, one or more AIDS prevention videotapes or films and supporting materials for teachers," and then goes on to call for other kinds of activities—including a parent meeting:

> It is the intent of the Legislature that, in addition
> to the viewing of the AIDS prevention videotape
> or film, local prevention instruction programs
> should include, to the extent local resources
> and time are available, at least the following
> activities to enhance the understanding of the

---

10. For more details on this exceptional program or complete information on conducting an AIDS Communication Conference (available on computer disk or hard copy for twenty-five dollars), write to Seattle–Kings County Chapter, American Red Cross, P.O. Box 24286, Seattle, WA 98124, Attention: Hope Tuttle, or phone 206-323-2345.

seriousness of the public health dangers of AIDS:

1. Appropriate classroom discussion.
2. Parent meeting.
3. Dissemination of the videotape or film for use by nonprofit community organizations.[11]

California State Senator Newton R. Russell was successful in amending Senator Hart's bill to require that the films, video, and other materials provided by the state should emphasize sexual abstinence as the primary method of AIDS protection.

That amendment of the legislation seems to have had one very significant impact:

There were two strong AIDS education videos on the market for use in schools.[12] In their original version, neither of them gave any significant place to abstinence. They seemed to presume sexual activity.

Shortly after Senator Hart's amended bill was passed out of committee, the producers of those videos announced that new versions would soon be available, and that these would *emphasize abstinence.*

Don't Settle for Too Little

The number of sexually active teens is *so high,* and the risk they face *so great,* that it is easy to settle for "safer

---

11. From the text of California State Senate Bill No. 136, 1987.
12. The cost of these videos would preclude their being purchased for home use.

sex" activities. Everything in our society points to this as the more realistic approach.

But every teen—and young adult, too—needs to know that it is okay to say no to sex outside of marriage, just as it is okay to say no to drugs, to alcohol, and to cigarettes.

Sex education classes must fully support those who decide to say no to sex. The teens in those classes must be told the truth—the whole truth—so that their decisions about sex can be well thought out. And those who choose to be active must know the risks and the protection available.

There is no easy answer to this sex/no sex war. The battle rages in the world of adults where often sex-with-whomever-I-want, whenever-I-want is treated as a right. How could we expect less of the young who follow so closely in our footsteps?

Parents *must* involve themselves in their children's sex education. Regardless of what you think about the sex/ health education or family life programs in your local schools, you must at least be a full participant in your children's sex education—at home *and* at school.

The Surgeon General has said that at home, "Parents can instill in their children their own moral and ethical standards." Almost one-half of America's concerned parents have never had as much as a single conversation with their teenagers about sexuality.

At school you can be a concerned friend, maintaining an ongoing supportive dialogue with school officials, and if possible, with the actual classroom teachers. Parents can be very vocal in their criticism of these programs. Few, if any, ever take the time to become knowledgeable and involved.

Talk of sex education raises parental concerns. The Surgeon General's hate mail makes that clear. But the specter of our current AIDS crisis *must* force us into a new era of reasoned, thoughtful cooperation among parents, teachers, and school officials.

In the height of the school prayer debate in the United States, a nationally known religious leader asked a large prayer breakfast audience, "How many of you are opposed to our children being denied the opportunity to be led in a prayer in school?"

Almost every hand in the audience was raised. Some even responded verbally.

Then the speaker quietly asked another question: "How many of you have prayed with your child some time this week?"

There was silence, and very few hands were raised.

We Are Responsible

Could it be that the sexual activity of our young is, at least in part, the result of a lack of open, frank, caring parental input?

Could it be that some of us fear the school's sex education voice, because our children have never heard our voice on the subject?

If we were to speak to our children about sexual activity—however timid our effort—doesn't it make sense to believe that our voice would be *at least* as respected as that of the schoolteacher?

At the very least, our compassionate concern that they say no to sex would compete strongly with the more permissive attitudes of some of their friends. As our young struggle to make their own difficult—and now very risky—decisions about sexual activity, they need the help of knowledgeable, patient parents.

You can protect yourself and your family from AIDS if you make the decision to do what must be done.

And the desire to protect your family can open the door to new understanding and fuller, more rewarding relationships.

Appendix A

Resources

For More Information on AIDS

National AIDS Hotline
Operated by the Public Health Service
1-800-342-AIDS

AIDS Education Fund
2335 18th Street, N.W.
Washington, D.C. 20039
202-332-5939

AIDS Action Council
729 8th Street, S.E., Suite 200
Washington, D.C. 20003
202-547-3101

United States Conference of Mayors
AIDS Information Exchange
1620 Eye Street, N.W.
Washington, D.C. 20006
202-293-7330

Minority Task Force on AIDS
c/o New York City Council of Churches
475 Riverside Drive, Room 456
New York, NY 10115
212-749-1214

Mothers of AIDS Patients (MAP)
c/o Barbara Peabody
3403 E Street
San Diego, CA 92102
619-234-3432

National Association of People with AIDS
P.O. Box 65472
Washington, D.C. 20035
202-483-7979

National Council of Churches/AIDS Task Force
475 Riverside Drive, Room 572
New York, NY 10115
212-870-2421

San Francisco AIDS Foundation
333 Valencia Street, 4th floor
San Francisco, CA 94103
415-863-2437

American Association of Physicians for Human Rights
P.O. Box 14366
San Francisco, CA 94114
415-558-9353

American Foundation for AIDS Research
9601 Wilshire Boulevard, Mezzanine
Los Angeles, CA 90210-5294
213-273-5547
   or
40 West 57th Street, Suite 406
New York, NY 10019-4001
212-333-3118

Hispanic AIDS Forum
c/o APRED
853 Broadway, Suite 2007
New York, NY 10003
212-870-1902 or 212-870-1864

Los Angeles AIDS Project
1362 Santa Monica Boulevard
Los Angeles, CA 90046
213-871-AIDS

For Information or Referrals in Canada

Canadian Public Health Association
1335 Carling Avenue
Ottawa, Canada K1Z 8N8
613-725-3769

National AIDS Centre
Health and Welfare Canada
Ottawa, Canada K1A 0L2
613-957-1772

Books and Reports

For a free copy of the
Surgeon General's Report on AIDS
write to:
AIDS
P.O. Box 14252
Washington, D.C. 20044
301-443-0292

Confronting AIDS: Directions for Public Health, Health Care, and Research
Prepared by the
Institutes of Medicine, National Academy of Sciences
National Academy Press
2101 Constitution Avenue, N.W.
Washington, D.C. 20418

What We Told Our Kids About Sex by Betsy A. Weisman
and Michael H. Weisman, M.D.
Published by Harcourt Brace Jovanovich.
  Helps preteens and their parents answer essential questions.

Appendix A

Pamphlets

A series of pamphlets jointly produced by the American Red
Cross and the United States Public Health Service:
  AIDS and Your Job: Are There Risks?
  AIDS, Sex and You
  Caring for the AIDS Patient at Home
  *AIDS and Children: Information for Teachers and
    School Officials*
  Gay and Bisexual Men and AIDS
  If Your Test for Antibodies to the AIDS Virus Is Positive
  Facts About AIDS and Drug Abuse

These pamphlets are available from your local chapter of the
American Red Cross or by writing:
American Red Cross
AIDS Education Office
1730 D Street, N.W.
Washington, D.C. 20006
202-737-8300

Teens and AIDS: Playing It Safe
(Sold in packets of 100 for $10.00.)
American Council of Life Insurance, Department 190
1001 Pennsylvania Avenue, N.W.
Washington, D.C. 20004-2599
202-624-2000

AIDS: What Young Adults Should Know
Instructor's Manual $8.95
Student's Guide $2.50
Published by American Alliance for Health,
Physical Education, Recreation, and Dance
1900 Association Drive
Reston, VA 22091
703-476-3400

Available in Canada from
Douglas and McIntyre Publishers
604-255-7701
(Also available in Spanish.)

Videos for School Use

(Should be previewed before showing.)
Drugs, Sex and AIDS
Narrated by Rae Dawn Chong
Available for purchase or rental from
O.D.N. Production
74 Varick Street, Suite 304
New York, NY 10013
212-431-8923
  and
AIDS
Hosted by Ally Sheedy
Available for purchase or rental from
Walt Disney Educational Media Company
Attention: Customer Service
10316 N.W. Prairie View Road
Kansas City, MO 64153-9990
800-423-2555
(Also available in filmstrip format.)

The Red Cross ARC/AIDS Prevention Program for Youth
includes *A Letter From Brian* (available for loan on film or
videotape), a teacher's guide, student workbook, and parent.
support brochure.
  Available from your local American Red Cross chapter.

AIDS Policies of Local Governments

For a review of actual policies instituted by local governments in the United States regarding AIDS in schools, the

workplace, and in other community situations, request a copy of *Local Policies in Response to AIDS, ARC and HIV Infection* from:

United States Conference of Mayors
1620 Eye Street, N.W.
Washington, D.C. 20006
　Price: $5.00

Personal Information

The AIDS Hotline in your community_____

_____

Your doctor_____

_____

Your state or local public health office_____

_____

Your local chapter of the American Red Cross_____

_____

Appendix B

Education and Foster Care of Children Infected with Human T-Lymphotropic Virus Type III/Lymphadenopathy-Associated Virus[1]

T he information and recommendations contained in this document were developed and compiled by CDC in consultation with individuals appointed by their organizations to represent the Conference of State and Territorial Epidemiologists, the Association of State and Territorial Health Officers, the National Association of County Health Officers, the Division of Maternal and Child Health (Health Resources and Services Administration), the National Association for Elementary School Principals, the National Association of State School Nurse Consultants, the National Congress of Parents and Teachers, and the Children's Aid Society. The consultants also included the mother of a child with acquired immunodeficiency syndrome (AIDS), a legal advisor to a state education department, and several pediatricians who are experts in the field of pediatric AIDS. This document is made available to assist state and local health and education departments in developing guidelines for their particular situations and locations.

---

1. Human T-lymphotropic virus III (HTLV-III) and lymphadenopathy-associated virus (LAV) are names for the AIDS virus referred to in this book as HIV.

These recommendations apply to all children known to be infected with human T-lymphotropic virus type III/lympha-denopathy-associated virus (HTLV-III/LAV). This includes children with AIDS as defined for reporting purposes (Table 1); children who are diagnosed by their physicians as having an illness due to infection with HTLV-III/LAV but who do not meet the case definition, and children who are asymptomatic but have virologic or serologic evidence of infection with HTLV-III/LAV. These recommendations do not apply to siblings of infected children unless they are also infected.

Background

The Scope of the Problem As of August 20, 1985, 183 of the 12,599 reported cases of AIDS in the United States were among children under 18 years of age. This number is expected to double in the next year. Children with AIDS have been reported from 23 states, the District of Columbia, and Puerto Rico, with 75% residing in New York, California, Florida, and New Jersey.

The 183 AIDS patients reported to CDC represent only the most severe form of HTLV-III/LAV infection, i.e., those children who develop opportunistic infections or malignancies (Table 1). As in adults with HTLV-III/LAV infection, many infected children may have milder illness or may be asymptomatic.

Legal Issues Among the legal issues to be considered in forming guidelines for the education and foster care of HTLV-III/LAV-infected children are the civil rights aspects of public school attendance, the protections for handicapped children under 20 U.S.C. 1401 et seq. and 29 U.S.C. 794, the confidentiality of a student's school record under state laws and under 20 U.S.C. 1232g, and employee right-to-know statutes for public employees in some states.

Confidentiality Issues The diagnosis of AIDS or associated illnesses evokes much fear from others in contact with the patient and may evoke suspicion of life styles that may not be acceptable to some persons. Parents of HTLV-III/LAV-infected

Table 1. Provisional care definition for acquired immunodeficiency syndrome (AIDS) surveillance of children

For the limited purposes of epidemiologic surveillance, CDC defines a case of pediatric acquired immunodeficiency syndrome (AIDS) as a child who has had:
1. A reliably diagnosed disease at least moderately indicative of underlying cellular immunodeficiency, and
2. No known cause of underlying cellular immunodeficiency or any other reduced resistance reported to be associated with that disease.

The diseases accepted as sufficiently indicative of underlying cellular immunodeficiency are the same as those used in defining AIDS in adults. In the absence of these opportunistic diseases, a histologically confirmed diagnosis of chronic lymphoid interstitial pneumonitis will be considered indicative of AIDS unless test(s) for HTLV-III/LAV are negative. Congenital infections, e.g., toxoplasmosis or herpes simplex virus infection in the first month after birth or cytomegalovirus infection in the first 6 months after birth must be excluded.

Specific conditions that must be excluded in a child are:
1. Primary immunodeficiency diseases—severe combined immuno-deficiency, DiGeorge syndrome, Wiskott-Aldrich syndrome, ataxia-telangiectasia, graft versus host disease, neutropenia, neutrophil function abnormality, agammaglobulinemia, or hypogam-maglobulinemia with raised IgM.
2. Secondary immunodeficiency associated with immunosuppressive therapy, lymphoreticular malignancy, or starvation.

children should be aware of the potential for social isolation should the child's condition become known to others in the care or educational setting. School, day-care, and social service personnel and others involved in educating and caring for these children should be sensitive to the need for confidentiality and the right to privacy in these cases.

Assessment of Risks
Risk Factors for Acquiring HTLV-III/LAV Infection and Transmission In adults and adolescents, HTLV-III/LAV is transmitted primarily through sexual contact (homosexual or heterosexual) and through parenteral exposure to infected blood or blood products. HTLV-III/LAV has been isolated from blood, semen, saliva, and tears but transmission has not been docu-

mented from saliva and tears. Adults at increased risk for acquiring HTLV-III/LAV include homosexual/bisexual men, intravenous drug abusers, persons transfused with contaminated blood or blood products, and sexual contacts of persons with HTLV-III/LAV infection or in groups at increased risk for infection.

The majority of infected children acquire the virus from their infected mothers in the perinatal period (1–4). In utero or intrapartum transmission are likely, and one child reported from Australia apparently acquired the virus postnatally, possibly from ingestion of breast milk (5). Children may also become infected through transfusion of blood or blood products that contain the virus. Seventy percent of the pediatric cases reported to CDC occurred among children whose parent had AIDS or was a member of a group at increased risk of acquiring HTLV-III/LAV infection, 20% of the cases occurred among children who had received blood or blood products, and for 10% investigations are incomplete.

Risk of Transmission in the School, Day-Care or Foster-Care Setting None of the identified cases of HTLV-III/LAV infection in the United States are known to have been transmitted in the school, day-care, or foster-care setting or through other casual person-to-person contact. Other than the sexual partners of HTLV-III/LAV-infected patients and infants born to infected mothers, none of the family members of the over 12,000 AIDS patients reported to CDC have been reported to have AIDS. Six studies of family members of patients with HTLV-III/LAV infection have failed to demonstrate HTLV-III/LAV transmission to adults who were not sexual contacts of the infected patients or to older children who were not likely at risk from perinatal transmission (6–11).

Based on current evidence, casual person-to-person contact as would occur among schoolchildren appears to pose no risk. However, studies of the risk of transmission through contact between younger children and neurologically handicapped children who lack control of their body secretions are very limited. Based on experience with other communicable diseases, a theoretical potential for transmission would be greatest among these children. It should be emphasized that any theoretical transmission would most likely involve exposure of open skin lesions or mucous membranes to blood and possibly other body fluids of an infected person.

Risks to the Child with HTLV-III/LAV Infection HTLV-III/LAV infection may result in immunodeficiency. Such children may have a greater risk of encountering infectious agents in a school or day-care setting than at home. Foster homes with multiple children may also increase the risk. In addition, younger children and neurologically handicapped children who may display behaviors such as mouthing of toys would be expected to be at greater risk for acquiring infections. Immunodepressed children are also at greater risk of suffering severe complications from such infections as chickenpox, cytomegalovirus, tuberculosis, herpes simplex, and measles. Assessment of the risk to the immunodepressed child is best made by the child's physician who is aware of the child's immune status. The risk of acquiring some infections, such as chickenpox, may be reduced by prompt use of specific immune globulin following a known exposure.

Recommendations

1. Decisions regarding the type of educational and care setting for HTLV-III/LAV-infected children should be based on the behavior, neurologic development, and physical condition of the child and the expected type of interaction with others in that setting. These decisions are best made using the team approach including the child's physician, public health personnel, the child's parent or guardian, and personnel associated with the proposed care or educational setting. In each case, risks

and benefits to both the infected child and to others in the setting should be weighed.

2. For most infected school-aged children, the benefits of an unrestricted setting would outweigh the risks of their acquiring potentially harmful infections in the setting and the apparent nonexistent risk of transmission of HTLV-III/LAV. These children should be allowed to attend school and after-school day-care and to be placed in a foster home in an unrestricted setting.

3. For the infected preschool-aged child and for some neurologically handicapped children who lack control of their body secretions or who display behavior, such as biting, and those children who have uncoverable, oozing lesions, a more restricted environment is advisable until more is known about transmission in these settings. Children infected with HTLV-III/LAV should be cared for and educated in settings that minimize exposure of other children to blood or body fluids.

4. Care involving exposure to the infected child's body fluids and excrement, such as feeding and diaper changing, should be performed by persons who are aware of the child's HTLV-III/LAV infection and the modes of possible transmission. In any setting involving an HTLV-III/LAV-infected person, good handwashing after exposure to blood and body fluids and before caring for another child should be observed, and gloves should be worn if open lesions are present on the caretaker's hands. Any open lesions on the infected person should also be covered.

5. Because other infections in addition to HTLV-III/LAV can be present in blood or body fluids, all schools and day-care facilities, regardless of whether children with HTLV-III/LAV infection are attending, should adopt routine procedures for ʰandling blood or body fluids. Soiled

surfaces should be promptly cleaned with disinfectants, such as household bleach (diluted 1 part bleach to 10 parts water). Disposable towels or tissues should be used whenever possible, and mops should be rinsed in the disinfectant. Those who are cleaning should avoid exposure of open skin lesions or mucous membranes to the blood or body fluids.

6. The hygienic practices of children with HTLV-III/LAV infection may improve as the child matures. Alternatively, the hygienic practices may deteriorate if the child's condition worsens. Evaluation to assess the need for a restricted environment should be performed regularly.

7. Physicians caring for children born to mothers with AIDS or at increased risk of acquiring HTLV-III/LAV infection should consider testing the children for evidence of HTLV-III/LAV infection for medical reasons. For example, vaccination of infected children with live virus vaccines, such as the measles-mumps-rubella vaccine (MMR), may be hazardous. These children also need to be followed closely for problems with growth and development and given prompt and aggressive therapy for infections and exposure to potentially lethal infections, such as varicella. In the event that an antiviral agent or other therapy for HTLV-III/LAV infection becomes available, these children should be considered for such therapy. Knowledge that a child is infected will allow parents and other caretakers to take precautions when exposed to the blood and body fluids of the child.

8. Adoption and foster-care agencies should consider adding HTLV-III/LAV screening to their routine medical evaluations of children at increased risk of infection before placement in the foster or adoptive home, since these parents must make decisions regarding the medi-

cal care of the child and must consider the possible social and psychological effects on their families.

9. Mandatory screening as a condition for school entry is not warranted based on available data.

10. Persons involved in the care and education of HTLV-III/LAV-infected children should respect the child's right to privacy, including maintaining confidential records. The number of personnel who are aware of the child's condition should be kept at a minimum needed to assure proper care of the child and to detect situations where the potential for transmission may increase (e.g., bleeding injury).

11. All educational and public health departments, regardless of whether HTLV-III/LAV-infected children are involved, are strongly encouraged to inform parents, children, and educators regarding HTLV-III/LAV and its transmission. Such education would greatly assist efforts to provide the best care and education for infected children while minimizing the risk of transmission to others.

This document is an excerpt from a report in the *Morbidity and Mortality Weekly Report*, August 30, 1985. For the complete set of recommendations, contact Department of Health and Human Services, Public Health Service, Centers for Disease Control, Atlanta, Georgia 30333.

For a simplified statement on this subject, request a copy of *AIDS and Children: Information for Teachers and School Officials* from your local chapter of the American Red Cross, or from the address listed in Appendix A.

For a review of actual policies instituted by local governments in the United States regarding AIDS in schools, the workplace, and in other community situations, request a copy of *Local Policies in Response to AIDS, ARC and HIV Infection* from the address listed in Appendix A.

Appendix C

Summary: Recommendations for Preventing Transmission of Infection with Human T-Lymphotropic Virus Type III/ Lymphadenopathy-Associated Virus[1] in the Workplace

The information and recommendations contained in this document have been developed with particular emphasis on health-care workers and others in related occupations in which exposure might occur to blood from persons infected with HTLV-III/LAV, the "AIDS virus." Because of public concern about the purported risk of transmission of HTLV-III/LAV by persons providing personal services and those preparing and serving food and beverages, this document also addresses personal-service and food-service workers. Finally, it addresses "other workers"—persons in settings such as offices, schools, factories, and construction sites, where there is no known risk of AIDS virus transmission.

Because AIDS is a bloodborne, sexually transmitted disease that is not spread by casual contact, this document does *not* recommend routine HTLV-III/LAV antibody screening for the groups addressed. Because AIDS is not transmitted through preparation or serving of food and beverages, these recommendations state that food-service workers known to be infected with AIDS should not be restricted from work unless they have

---

1. Human T-lymphotropic virus III (HTLV-III) and lymphadenopathy-associated virus (LAV) are names for the AIDS virus referred to in this book as HIV.

another infection or illness for which such restriction would be warranted.

This document contains detailed recommendations for precautions appropriate to prevent transmission of all bloodborne infectious diseases to people exposed—in the course of their duties—to blood from persons who may be infected with HTLV-III/LAV. They emphasize that health-care workers should take all possible precautions to prevent needlestick injury. The recommendations are based on the well-documented modes of HTLV-III/LAV transmission and incorporate a "worst case" scenario, the hepatitis B model of transmission. Because the hepatitis B virus is also bloodborne and is both hardier and more infectious than HTLV-III/LAV, recommendations that would prevent transmission of hepatitis B will also prevent transmission of AIDS.

Formulation of specific recommendations for health-care workers who perform invasive procedures is in progress.

Recommendations for Preventing Transmission of Infection With Human T-Lymphotropic Virus Type III/ Lymphadenopathy-Associated Virus in the Workplace

Persons at increased risk of acquiring infection with human T-lymphotropic virus type III/lymphadenopathy-associated virus (HTLV-III/LAV), the virus that causes acquired immunodeficiency syndrome (AIDS), include homosexual and bisexual men, intravenous (IV) drug abusers, persons transfused with contaminated blood or blood products, heterosexual contacts of persons with HTLV-III/LAV infection, and children born to infected mothers. HTLV-III/LAV is transmitted through sexual contact, parenteral exposure to infected blood or blood components, and perinatal transmission from mother to neonate. HTLV-III/LAV has been isolated from blood, semen, saliva, tears, breast milk, and urine and is likely to be isolated from some other body fluids, secretions, and excretions, but epidemiologic evidence has implicated only blood and semen in transmission. Studies of nonsexual household contacts of AIDS patients indicate that casual contact with saliva and tears does not result in transmission of infection. Spread of infection to household contacts of infected persons has not been detected when the household contacts have not been sex partners or have not been infants of infected mothers. The kind of nonsexual person-to-person contact that generally occurs among workers and clients or consumers in the workplace does not pose a risk for transmission of HTLV-III/LAV.

As in the development of any such recommendations, the paramount consideration is the protection of the public's health. The following recommendations have been developed for all workers, particularly workers in occupations in which exposure might occur to blood from individuals infected with HTLV-III/LAV. These recommendations reinforce and supplement the specific recommendations that were published earlier for clinical and laboratory staffs (1) and for dental-care personnel and persons performing necropsies and morticians' services (2). Because of public concern about the purported risk of transmission of HTLV-III/LAV by persons providing personal services and by food and beverages, these recommendations contain information and recommendations for personal-service and food-service workers. Finally, these recommendations address workplaces in general where there is no known risk of transmission of HTLV-III/LAV (e.g., offices, schools, factories, construction sites). Formulation of specific recommendations for health-care workers (HCWs) who perform invasive procedures (e.g., surgeons, dentists) is in progress. Separate recommendations are also being developed to prevent HTLV-III/LAV transmission in prisons, other correctional facilities, and institutions housing individuals who may exhibit uncontrollable behavior (e.g., custodial institutions) and in the perinatal setting. In addition, separate recommendations have already been developed for children in schools and day-care centers (3).

HTLV-III/LAV-infected individuals include those with AIDS (4), those diagnosed by their physician(s) as having other illnesses due to infection with HTLV-III/LAV, and those who have virologic or serologic evidence of infection with HTLV-III/LAV but who are not ill.

Considerations Relevant to Other Workers

Personal-Service Workers (PSWs) PSWs are defined as individuals whose occupations involve close personal contact with clients (e.g., hairdressers, barbers, estheticians, cosmetologists, manicurists, pedicurists, massage therapists). PSWs whose services (tattooing, ear piercing, acupuncture, etc.) require needles or other instruments that penetrate the skin should follow precautions indicated for HCWs. Although there is no evidence of transmission of HTLV-III/LAV from clients to PSWs, from PSWs to clients, or between clients of PSWs, a risk of transmission would exist from PSWs to clients and vice versa in situations where there is both (1) trauma to one of the individuals that would provide a portal of entry for the virus and (2) access of blood or serous fluid from one infected person to the open tissue of the other, as could occur if either sustained a cut. A risk of transmission from client to client exists when instruments contaminated with blood are not sterilized or disinfected between clients. However, HBV transmission has been documented only rarely in acupuncture, ear piercing, and tattoo establishments and never in other personal-service settings, indicating that any risk for HTLV-III/LAV transmission in personal-service settings must be extremely low.

All PSWs should be educated about transmission of blood-borne infections, including HTLV-III/LAV and HBV. Such education should emphasize principles of good hygiene, antisepsis, and disinfection. This education can be accomplished by national or state professional organizations, with assistance from state and local health departments, using lectures at meetings or self-instructional materials. Licensure requirements should include evidence of such education. Instruments that are intended to penetrate the skin (e.g., tattooing and acupuncture needles, ear piercing devices) should be used once and disposed of or be thoroughly cleaned and sterilized after each use using procedures recommended for use in health-care institutions. Instruments not intended to penetrate the skin but which may become contaminated with blood (e.g., razors), should be used for only one client and be disposed of or thoroughly cleaned and disinfected after use using procedures recommended for use in health-care institutions. Any PSW with exudative lesions or weeping dermatitis, regardless of HTLV-III/LAV infection status, should refrain from direct contact with clients until the condition resolves. PSWs known to be infected with HTLV-III/LAV need not be restricted from work unless they have evidence of other infections or illnesses for which any PSW should also be restricted.

Routine serologic testing of PSWs for antibody to HTLV-III/LAV is not recommended to prevent transmission from PSWs to clients.

Food-Service Workers (FSWs) FSWs are defined as individuals whose occupations involve the preparation or serving of food or beverages (e.g., cooks, caterers, servers, waiters, bartenders, airline attendants). All epidemiologic and laboratory evidence indicates that bloodborne and sexually transmitted infections are not transmitted during the preparation or serving of food or beverages, and no instances of HBV or HTLV-III/LAV transmission have been documented in this setting.

All FSWs should follow recommended standards and practices of good personal hygiene and food sanitation (26). All FSWs should exercise care to avoid injury to hands when preparing food. Should such an injury occur, both aesthetic and sanitary considerations would dictate that food contaminated with blood be discarded. FSWs known to be infected with HTLV-III/LAV need not be restricted from work unless

189

they have evidence of other infection or illness for which any FSW should also be restricted.

Routine serologic testing of FSWs for antibody to HTLV-III/LAV is not recommended to prevent disease transmission from FSWs to consumers.

Other Workers Sharing the Same Work Environment No known risk of transmission to co-workers, clients, or consumers exists from HTLV-III/LAV-infected workers in other settings (e.g., offices, schools, factories, construction sites). This infection is spread by sexual contact with infected persons, injection of contaminated blood or blood products, and by perinatal transmission. Workers known to be infected with HTLV-III/LAV should not be restricted from work solely based on this finding. Moreover, they should not be restricted from using telephones, office equipment, toilets, showers, eating facilities, and water fountains. Equipment contaminated with blood or other body fluids of any worker, regardless of HTLV-III/LAV infection status, should be cleaned with soap and water or a detergent. A disinfectant solution or a fresh solution of sodium hypochlorite (household bleach, see above) should be used to wipe the area after cleaning.

Other Issues in the Workplace

The information and recommendations contained in this document do not address all the potential issues that may have to be considered when making specific employment decisions for persons with HTLV-III/LAV infection. The diagnosis of HTLV-III/LAV infection may evoke unwarranted fear and suspicion in some co-workers. Other issues that may be considered include the need for confidentiality, applicable federal, state, or local laws governing occupational safety and health, civil rights of employees, workers' compensation laws, provisions of collective bargaining agreements, confidentiality of medical records, informed consent, employee and patient privacy rights, and employee right-to-know statutes.

Development of These Recommendations

The information and recommendations contained in these recommendations were developed and compiled by CDC and other PHS agencies in consultation with individuals representing various organizations. The following organizations were represented: Association of State and Territorial Health Officials, Conference of State and Territorial Epidemiologists, Association of State and Territorial Public Health Laboratory Directors, National Association of County Health Officials, American Hospital Association, United States Conference of Local Health Officers, Association for Practitioners in Infection Control, Society of Hospital Epidemiologists of America, American Dental Association, American Medical Association, American Nurses' Association, American Association of Medical Colleges, American Association of Dental Schools, National Institutes of Health, Food and Drug Administration, Food Research Institute, National Restaurant Association, National Hairdressers and Cosmetologists Association, National Gay Task Force, National Funeral Directors and Morticians Association, American Association of Physicians for Human Rights, and National Association of Emergency Medical Technicians. The consultants also included a labor union representative, an attorney, a corporate medical director, and a pathologist. However, these recommendations may not reflect the views of individual consultants or the organizations they represented.

This document is an excerpt from a report in the *Morbidity and Mortality Weekly Report*, November 15, 1985. For the complete recommendations contact Department of Health and Human Services, Public Health Service, Centers for Disease Control, Atlanta, Georgia 30333.

For a simplified statement on this subject, request a copy of *AIDS and Your Job: Are There Risks?* from your local chapter of the American Red Cross or from the address listed in Appendix A.

191